HEALING YOUR
CHRONIC-ILLNESS
GRIEF

Also by Dr. Alan Wolfelt

Grief One Day at a Time:
365 Meditations to Help You Heal After Loss

Healing the Adult Child's Grieving Heart:
100 Practical Ideas After Your Parent Dies

Healing the Adult Sibling's Grieving Heart:
100 Practical Ideas After Your Brother or Sister Dies

Healing Your Grief About Aging:
100 Practical Ideas on Growing Older with
Confidence, Meaning, and Grace

The Mourner's Book of Hope:
30 Days of Inspiration

Understanding Your Grief:
Ten Essential Touchstones for Finding Hope and Healing Your Heart

When Your Pet Dies:
A Guide to Mourning, Remembering, and Healing

The Wilderness of Grief:
Finding Your Way

*Companion Press is dedicated to the education
and support of both the bereaved and bereavement
caregivers. We believe that those who companion
the bereaved by walking with them as they journey
in grief have a wondrous opportunity: to help others
embrace and grow through grief—and to lead
fuller, more deeply lived lives themselves
because of this important ministry.*

Companion
PRESS

For a complete catalog and ordering information, write or call:

Companion Press
The Center for Loss and Life Transition
3735 Broken Bow Road
Fort Collins, CO 80526
(970) 226-6050
www.centerforloss.com

HEALING YOUR CHRONIC-ILLNESS GRIEF

•

100 PRACTICAL IDEAS FOR LIVING YOUR BEST LIFE

•

JAIMIE A. WOLFELT
ALAN D. WOLFELT, PH.D.

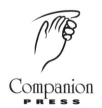

Companion
PRESS

Fort Collins, Colorado
An imprint of the Center for Loss and Life Transition

Companion Press is an imprint of the
Center for Loss and Life Transition
3735 Broken Bow Road
Fort Collins, Colorado 80526
www.centerforloss.com

26 25 24 23 22 21 20 19   5 4 3 2 1

ISBN 978-1617222771

To all the people with chronic illnesses that have been willing to teach us about their experience so we could pen this book in an effort to help others.

Thank you.

CONTENTS

INTRODUCTION

Welcome to this book and this conversation. What an honor to have you.

Of course, perhaps like you, we wish there weren't a need for such a book. We wish our lives weren't encumbered with chronic illness. We wish you weren't chronically ill. Please know that we have deep empathy for you and for the many losses chronic illness may have brought into your life.

At the same time, we are grateful for this opportunity to shine some light into the darkness. We are proud to be the bearers of hope, which is an expectation of a good that is yet to be. We're honored to walk alongside you in your chronic-illness journey and hold that light of hope high.

Yes, our commitment to you is that you will feel hopeful as you read this resource. While we don't know the specific details of your unique experience with chronic illness, we want you to know: you are not alone. The ability to survive and thrive comes in supporting each other and having gratitude for life, living, and loving.

Why we wrote this book

It all started about a month before my (Jaimie's) tenth birthday. I remember telling my mom, who is a primary care physician, that I had been going to the bathroom a lot. I also seemed to be in a really bad mood all of the time. My mom took me into her office for a urine test. After calling my pediatrician about the test results, Mom took me to the emergency room. I didn't know what was wrong but I was extremely scared. I remember taking my favorite stuffed animal, Perkins, with me to the hospital where I was diagnosed with Type 1 diabetes.

I don't have very many memories about being in the hospital. I stayed for a few days while they helped my blood sugar get back in range and educated us about what Type 1 diabetes was. I did not really understand what was happening or what diabetes was. I remember after I got home that I didn't want to take the insulin shots. I remember crying; I didn't understand why this had happened to me and why I would have to keep taking shots. I also remember my mom and dad consoling me and crying with me. We were all grieving the life I had before diabetes and the challenges I would face in the future with diabetes.

It has been fourteen years since I was diagnosed with diabetes. Although there have been many challenges along the way, I am happy to say that I now live a happy and full life with Type 1 diabetes. Every day I must live with the awareness that I have a chronic illness—a potentially dangerous illness that requires constant monitoring and can lead to permanent physical damage, painful and limiting side effects, and even a foreshortened life. Some days are harder than others, some hours are harder than others, some weeks or months are harder than others, but I have the resources to create a healthy and full life while managing my diabetes. I still grieve some of the aspects and challenges that come along with diabetes, but I am thankful for my health and the things that diabetes has brought into my life.

As it happens, my dad and coauthor of this book, Dr. Alan Wolfelt, is a world-renowned grief counselor, author, and speaker. His passion is helping people understand their natural and necessary grief after life losses and find ways to mourn, or express, that grief so they can continue forward to live their best lives. It might seem odd to some of you to have a father who constantly talks about things like grief, death, and funerals, but to me, it's normal. In fact, I grew up just a few steps away from the Center for Loss and Life Transition. And my dad is far from morbid. He's actually really energetic, happy, and life-loving. He just knows that it's essential to intentionally acknowledge and embrace our grief as part of living with meaning, purpose, and yes, joy.

My dad (who also has severe chronic osteoarthritis and is a cancer survivor) has written many books on grief, mourning, and healing, so when he suggested to me that he and I write a book together about chronic-illness grief, I jumped at the chance. You see, I've found my own passion in the last few years, and it's helping others, especially children, with Type 1 diabetes cope with the emotional and social aspects of their disease. Right now I'm finishing my master's in counseling psychology and working at the Barbara Davis Center for Diabetes, which specializes in Type 1 research and care for both children and adults. Creating a grief-aware book on living well with chronic illness—something that could help me as well as you and potentially many others—seemed like a meaningful next step in my journey.

That's enough about me. Now let's talk about you.

The invisible epidemic of chronic illness

It often helps those of us with chronic illness to understand that we are not alone. Far from it, in fact. Six in ten Americans have a chronic disease, and four in ten have two or more chronic illnesses. Men and women of all ages are affected, children through seniors.

Among the most common are heart disease, autoimmune diseases, cancer, lung diseases, stroke, Alzheimer's, diabetes, kidney disease, and mental illness. Within each of these categories fall a number of specific illnesses. Chronic heart conditions range from coronary-artery disease to valve defects and arrhythmias, for example. And autoimmune diseases include conditions as diverse as Crohn's, asthma, multiple sclerosis, fibromyalgia, and lupus, just to name a few. Some chronic illnesses are considered congenital, such as hemophilia, Huntington's disease, and cystic fibrosis, while others, like rheumatoid arthritis, and Parkinson's disease, are more often developed over time.

What is your chronic illness, and what are your current challenges and fears regarding your illness? Please share them here:

_____

_____

_____

_____

So we come to this book with a vast variety of different backgrounds. Every chronic illness has unique symptoms, courses, degree of severity, treatments, and prognoses. Yet those of us who are affected by chronic illness also have a lot in common. We have a disease that is not going away—maybe for a while, maybe never. We share similar losses and experiences. We grieve our diminishments, pains, and limitations. For many of us, our illnesses and daily struggles may be largely invisible, but in the privacy of our own homes and hearts, we are unified in our desire to be seen, understood, supported, and loved.

We also want to live as well and as long as we can.

Whatever your illness and prognosis, we welcome you to this conversation. Thank you for joining us in exploring this important topic and finding ways to live our best lives.

Living well with chronic illness

This book is about two things: acknowledging, embracing, and expressing the normal and necessary grief of chronic illness, and living our best lives with chronic illness. You might think the two are mutually exclusive, but they're not. They actually go hand in hand.

Just as our chronic illnesses are part of who we are, our grief is part of who we are. People tend to think of grief as temporary, but it's not. Whenever we grieve a significant, life-altering loss, our grief is lifelong. When that loss goes on and on, building upon itself over time—as it often does with chronic illness—our grief may also be chronic. My dad has helped me understand that this is often referred to as chronic sorrow.

But even as we grieve, mourn, and deal with our chronic illnesses, we can also, at the same time, strive to live our best lives. We can live with intention and purpose. We can proactively seek meaning, peace, and joy.

And there are so many of us out there; we need not walk alone.

How to use this book

As promised, this book contains 100 ideas to help you acknowledge, embrace, and mourn your chronic-illness grief and live your best life despite the chronic illness and the chronic grief. Some of the ideas will teach you about principles of grief and mourning. The remainder will offer practical, here-and-now, action-oriented suggestions for embracing your grief, practicing self-care and self-compassion, and living out your hopes and dreams.

Some of the ideas will speak to your unique experiences more than others. If you come to an idea that doesn't seem to fit you, simply ignore it and turn to another page.

As you flip through these pages, you will also see that each idea includes a "Carpe Diem," which means, as fans of the movie *Dead Poets Society* will remember, "seize the day." Our hope is that you not relegate this resource to your shelves but instead keep it handy on your nightstand or desk. Pick it up often and turn to any page; the Carpe Diem suggestion might help you seize the day by giving you an exercise, action, or thought to consider today, right now, right this minute.

Please understand that nothing in this book should be construed as medical advice. If you have questions or concerns about any medical matter, you should consult your doctor or other healthcare provider. You should never delay seeking medical advice, disregard medical advice, or discontinue medical treatment because of ideas presented in this resource.

Thank you for picking up this book. We wish you courage, grace, comfort, and hope as you begin to explore this resource. We hope you will view this little book as an encouraging but bold friend who takes your hand and walks with you, by your side. As good friends do, let it fill you with the strength and belief that you can live well with chronic illness and continue to discover new meaning and purpose in your life.

Godspeed. We hope to meet you one day.

Jaimie Wolfelt   *Alan D. Wolfelt*

March 2019

1.

LEARN ABOUT YOUR DIAGNOSIS (AND EDUCATE OTHERS)

"Each patient carries his own doctor inside. They come to us now knowing this truth. We are at our best when they give the doctor who resides within each patient a chance to go to work."
— Dr. Albert Schweitzer

• If you're educated about your diagnosis and treatment options, you're in a much better position to advocate for your best care and live your best life.

• Read up on your symptoms and diagnosis. Learn about your treatment options, both traditional and non-traditional. Work to understand and keep track of your healthcare costs and insurance limitations. And when you're meeting with providers, don't be afraid to ask questions and seek second opinions.

• Come up with simple, clear ways to educate friends and family about your illness. Unless they're interested, you don't need to go into extensive detail, but it is helpful for them to know what you are experiencing and how it affects your life. It's also a good idea to let friends and family know about the small ways in which they can help or support you with your illness.

• Of course, there's a difference between being knowledgeable about your illness and *being* your illness. Some people with chronic illness develop a self-identity that is all about the illness. When this happens, the person's life becomes wholly defined by the illness. Yes, there is power and meaning in knowledge, participation, and advocacy. But whenever any one thing takes over a person's self-identity—be it a career, a relationship, a cause, or anything else—that person is usually putting up walls that cut them off from a whole, full life.

CARPE DIEM

What questions or doubts do you have about your diagnosis or symptoms? Do some reading today, or reach out to your healthcare provider.

2.

CLAIM YOUR ROLE AS EXPERT OF YOUR EXPERIENCE

*"Behind every chronic illness is just a person
trying to find their way in the world."*
— Glenn Schweitzer

- Do you find that lots of other people try to tell you what to do about your chronic illness?

- Eat this, not that. Go to this specialist. Try this miracle cure. Don't take that medication. Eliminate this, add that, read this. These people usually mean well, but they can be bossy sometimes—and outright ignorant at other times. Even different healthcare providers will offer up a wide variety of differing recommendations.

- Accurate information is a good thing, and being open to new ideas is also important, but you are the only one who can ultimately decide what's right for your body today, tomorrow, and the day after that.

- Your life isn't a democracy; it's a monarchy. When it comes to your life, you wear the crown. Wear it with pride and without apology.

CARPE DIEM
The next time someone tells you what to do about your
chronic illness, remember who's king or queen.

3.

TAKE CARE OF YOURSELF PHYSICALLY

"Take care of your body. It's the only place you have to live."
— Jim Rohn

- When it comes to chronic illness, this is a big one. We can't completely control our bodies, but we can and must take care of them. And when we take the best care of our bodies that we can, we are setting ourselves up for the best life experience we can.

- Keeping current with doctor and other health-provider appointments is essential. They are our team members, and we need their help staying on top of our health. This includes any holistic therapies that we have found help us.

- Eating nourishing food and drinking plenty of water is another baseline must. As the saying goes, garbage in, garbage out. Good nutrition has been proven to lessen inflammation (a contributor to many illnesses), stave off many common chronic conditions, and improve mood.

- Good sleep is as important as good diet. Optimizing our sleep habits and getting help from our health care providers or a sleep specialist when needed will ensure we feel our best.

- Gentle exercise that accommodates and respects our chronic conditions is the final cornerstone of responsible physical self-care. Life is motion, and our bodies function best when they move to the extent that they are able. A physical therapist or exercise specialist can help us create an exercise plan that works for us.

CARPE DIEM

Have you seen a nutritionist? Many insurances cover nutrition consultations. It's a great way to affirm that you're giving your body the macro- and micronutrients it needs.

4.

NURTURE SELF-COMPASSION

"The truth is we're all a little bit broken.
We must learn to love the broken pieces of ourselves—
be gentle and empathetic with ourselves and others."

— Karen Salmansohn

- You are the expert of your own experience. No one else can live inside your consciousness or body. No one else can experience your life as you do.

- While we hope others can and will strive to understand and empathize (more on that later), you are at the helm of your life. You are the captain of your own ship.

- You have the greatest potential to offer yourself self-understanding and self-empathy. Self-compassion includes the ways that you speak to yourself with your inner voice every day about your chronic illness. Be self-compassionate on the hard days, and give yourself permission to embrace the reality that not every day will be perfect.

- Just as it is a choice for those around you, it is a choice for you to treat yourself either with disregard or regard, disdain or empathy, carelessness or compassion.

- Nurturing self-compassion means to consciously and proactively choose, over and over, in big ways and small, to take care of yourself, forgive yourself when necessary, and love yourself.

- Whenever you choose self-compassion, you are choosing hope, love, and life.

CARPE DIEM
Right now, offer yourself a gift of self-compassion.
Speak words of kindness to yourself, or choose to nurture
yourself in some small way, right this minute.

5.

BREATHE

- Mindful breathing is a super-simple practice that has the power to get us through and beyond almost any challenging moment.

- Just stop whatever it is you're doing, sit comfortably, and close your eyes. Now concentrate on your breath.

- Breathe in slowly through your nose, and exhale slowly through your mouth. As you're doing so, consciously relax all the muscles in your body.

- When thoughts come, set them aside and return your awareness to your breath and the rise and fall of your belly and your chest. If counting helps you stay focused on your breath, silently count 1-2-3-4 as you inhale and 1-2-3-4 as you exhale.

- When you're stressed, try mindful breathing for one minute. As you get better at it, you can build to five or ten minutes, but you can also continue to turn to one-minute mindful breathing sessions when you need a quick reset.

CARPE DIEM
Put this book down and practice mindful
breathing for at least one minute.

6.

UNDERSTAND THE SIX NEEDS OF MOURNING

Need 1: Acknowledge the reality of your diagnosis and prognosis

"There is only one cardinal rule: One must always listen to the patient."
— Oliver Sacks

- You have a chronic illness. This can be a difficult reality to accept. Yet you must embrace this reality, bit by bit, day by day.

- If you are in the early weeks or months of your chronic-illness journey, you may still be struggling to accept this reality. It's common for this need of mourning to take a while. You will first acknowledge the reality of your illness with your head. Only over time will you come to acknowledge it with your heart.

- If, on the other hand, you are many months or years into your chronic-illness journey, you have probably come to acknowledge this reality. You have probably learned to live with your illness's demands and challenges.

- Growing comfortable with speaking the words aloud may help you with this mourning need. Learning to say, "I have _____" to friends, family members, and even strangers when the need arises will help you come to terms with the reality of your diagnosis and prognosis.

- At times you may push away the reality of your illness. It's normal to want to take breaks from the reality. Allow yourself these natural moments of temporary reprieve as well.

CARPE DIEM
Tell someone new about your illness today—maybe someone you've been meaning to tell.

7.

UNDERSTAND THE SIX NEEDS OF MOURNING

Need 2: Embrace the pain of your losses

"So, this is my life. And I want you to know that I am both happy and sad, and I'm still trying to figure out how that could be."
— Stephen Chbosky

- This need requires those of us with chronic illness to embrace the pain of any losses that stem from the illness—something we naturally would rather not do. It is easier to avoid, repress, or push away the pain. It is in embracing our normal and necessary grief, however, that we learn to reconcile ourselves to it.

- In the early weeks and months after our diagnoses, the pain of our current and potential future losses may be especially intense. We may think about the losses all the time. When we are in this phase, taking breaks from our normal and necessary pain is essential. It's healthy to distract ourselves with entertainment and conversations with friends and family about other things.

- Despite what you may have heard, embracing emotional and spiritual pain is not "feeling sorry for yourself." Instead, it is being honest about what you are thinking and feeling.

- While you do need to embrace the pain, you can only do it in doses, over time. It's healthy to alternate essential encountering of the pain with equally essential times of recreation and pleasure.

CARPE DIEM

Set aside half an hour today to sit with the pain of your losses.

8.

UNDERSTAND THE SIX NEEDS OF MOURNING

Need 3: Remember your past

"You must listen to the music of the past to sing in the present and dance into the future."

— Dr. Alan Wolfelt

- Your life story begins the day you are born and ends the day you die. (If you believe in an afterlife, a new story will begin then.)

- Have you always had your chronic illness? If not, your life story began before the onset of symptoms or your diagnosis. Yes, the illness is now part of your life story, but remembering your past makes hoping for your future possible.

- The onset of chronic illness can be a wake-up call. To embrace how it fits into your life and to consider what your life is all about, you must take time to reflect on your life so far. Who are you? What made you who you are? Which experiences and relationships have most shaped you?

- Your life is a story. Try telling the story of your whole life, from birth to this moment. Write it down, or tell it to someone else. The process of telling the story of your life has the power to help you integrate your chronic illness into a coherent narrative—a story that has shape, meaning, and purpose.

- As you remember your past, stop to linger on people, moments, and events for whom or which you are grateful. Express your gratitude in some way as you uncover these memories. Write a thank-you note, celebrate an *aha!*, or share a special memory with someone you know will appreciate it.

CARPE DIEM
Today, make a call or write a note of thanks to someone who helped shape your early life in positive ways.

9.

UNDERSTAND THE SIX NEEDS OF MOURNING

Need 4: Incorporate your illness into your self-identity

*"Chronic illness is hard. Pain is hard. Isolation is hard.
The financial cost is hard. Grieving is hard and necessary and
sometimes takes far longer than we ever imagined."*
— Cindee Snider

- You have a chronic illness. Coming to terms with the fact that you are someone who is ill is one of your needs of mourning.

- Chronic illness typically feels scary and bad. While you might eventually feel that your illness is something that has given you gifts, you probably wish it wasn't the price you had to pay for these gifts. In short, your chronic illness is a part of your self-identity, even if you wish it weren't.

- Whether you like it or not, somewhere along the way chronic illness became a significant part of your life's journey. Like other life challenges, such as a history of abuse or a disability, your chronic illness is one aspect of who you are. No, your chronic illness does not define you. But it is part of who you have become. Incorporating this reality into your self-identity is often arduous, painful work that takes a long time.

- While you must work through this difficult need yourself, know that many people with chronic illnesses ultimately learn to not only accept but embrace this new part of themselves.

CARPE DIEM
Find a blank piece of paper. This paper represents your entire self.
Now draw and label shapes on the paper that represent different
aspects of who you are. Make each shape proportionate
in size to its importance to your self-identity.
How large is the shape that represents your chronic illness?

10.

UNDERSTAND THE SIX NEEDS OF MOURNING

Need 5: Search for meaning

"Surrender is an incredibly difficult topic in light of chronic illness, because loss is often continued and sustained."

— Cindee Snider

- When we begin to experience symptoms or are diagnosed with a chronic illness, we may naturally also begin to question the meaning and purpose of life and death.

- "Why" questions may surface uncontrollably and often precede "How" questions. "Why did this have to happen?" and "Why me?" come before "How will I handle and live with this condition?"

- Sometimes we are taught not to ask why. We may be told asking why doesn't do us any good. Yet it is natural to ask why and search for meaning.

- You will almost certainly question your philosophy of life and explore religious or spiritual values as you work on this need.

- Remember that having faith or spirituality does not negate your need to mourn. Even if you believe that things happen for a reason or that there is a higher power in charge, your one-and-only life has been altered in challenging, painful ways by chronic illness. It's normal to feel dumbfounded and angry at a God whom you may feel has permitted such a thing to happen.

CARPE DIEM

What is the biggest "why?" question you have right now?
Talk about it with a good-listener friend today.

11.

UNDERSTAND THE SIX NEEDS OF MOURNING

Need 6: Receive ongoing support from others

"It got worse still as time went on because people did not sympathize with you anymore. They couldn't do enough for you at first, and that helped, and then they got bored with your troubles. But your troubles went on just the same, and you had to bear them alone."

— Elizabeth Goudge

- As human beings, we need the support of others when we are experiencing pain and loss.

- Don't feel ashamed of your dependence on others. If you are experiencing physical challenges, you may need a lot of help. You may need someone to take you to and from appointments and to accompany you to treatment sessions. You may need help running errands, doing laundry, caring for children, or paying bills. You also need moral and emotional support. Don't feel bad about this. Instead, take comfort knowing that others care.

- Unfortunately, our society places too much value on "carrying on" and "doing well." So, many people with chronic illness are abandoned by friends and family not long after diagnosis. We hope this did not happen to you, but if it did, know that many people with chronic illness share your experience.

- Others with chronic illness can be an excellent source of social, emotional, and spiritual support. They "get it." Consider joining a support group.

- Sometimes when you've had a chronic illness for a long time, friends and family may forget that you still need help. It's OK to remind them that because you have ongoing grief and challenges, you need ongoing support.

- If you are not getting the support from others that you need, please, ask for it. Usually people are more than willing to support you—they just need help understanding how they can help.

CARPE DIEM
Today, tell someone at least one concrete way they can support you in your chronic illness.

12.

MOURN "BEFORE"

*"Please be patient with me. Sometimes when I'm quiet, it's because
I need to figure myself out. It's not because I don't want to talk.
Sometimes there are no words for my thoughts."*

— Kamla Bolaños

- If you remember your life before you began to experience or were diagnosed with your chronic illness, you have a "before."

- "Before" often has the golden quality of nostalgic memory. "Before" was simpler, vaster, more hopeful. Everything was possible "before."

- Those of us with chronic illness often long for "before"—even if our memories of it are overly rose-colored. It's natural to yearn for the health and unadulterated happiness we remember.

- If we're missing "before," that means it's a loss for us, and that means we need to mourn it. We can mourn it by sharing our thoughts and feelings about "before" with others, or by journaling, creating art, or simply by immersing ourselves in memories and having a good cry.

- When we actively mourn "before," we're integrating it into our forward lives. We're not forgetting it. Instead, we're honoring it even as we learn to place more emphasis on creating meaning and purpose in our "after" lives today.

CARPE DIEM
Today, find a way to actively mourn some aspect of your "before."

13.

ACKNOWLEDGE ANY LOST HOPES AND DREAMS

"Picking up the pieces of a shattered dream is better than having no pieces to pick up at all."

— Matshona Dhliwayo

- Chronic illness presents us with many forks in the road, but some of those forks are bigger than others.

- Sometimes we may be brought to a fork in the road where we desperately want to choose one way but are forced to choose the other.

- Some of us would love to have children but cannot, for example. Others of us might have had dreams of traveling the world, attaining a challenging career, or achieving physical feats, but these dreams may have been rendered impossible by our illnesses.

- Sometimes our hearts break when we think about the futures we have lost. We might be tempted to not think about such things. We might prefer to deny our true feelings or distract ourselves from them. But denial and distraction don't help us forge new hopes and dreams.

- Actively mourning lost hopes and dreams helps us accommodate them. Talking about them with others is one effective way. Attending a support group is another. Writing about them in a journal is a third.

CARPE DIEM

Make time to actively mourn one of your lost hopes or dreams today.

14.

ACKNOWLEDGE THE GRIEF OF FRIENDS AND FAMILY

"There are three needs of the griever: To find the words for the loss, to say the words aloud, and to know that the words have been heard."

— Victoria Alexander

- We are not the only ones who grieve the losses we experience as a result of our illnesses. Those who love us grieve as well.

- The people who care about us also have a wide variety of thoughts and feelings about our conditions. Some may feel angry on our behalf. Some may be anxious about what the future holds. Others may feel sad about any limitations or pain we experience. Still others may feel guilty that they are well and we are not. All of these feelings (and more) are normal and natural. As Jaimie's father, I (Alan) experienced significant grief when she was diagnosed and continue to grieve for her challenging present and future.

- One of the best ways to cope with grief is to be open and honest about what you are feeling inside. You can help your friends and family members by modeling your own genuine mourning and by actively listening and empathizing when they express their thoughts and feelings.

- Sometimes, especially at times of crisis in the course of an illness, we may understandably be too consumed by our own physical symptoms and grief to attend to the grief of others. When this happens, it's healthy to set boundaries and to let our loved ones know that while we empathize with them, we are too overwhelmed right now to give them our full attention. We can encourage them to share their grief with others for the time being.

CARPE DIEM
Who else is grieving the repercussions of your chronic illness?
Acknowledge their grief in some small way today.

15.

TELL YOUR STORY

"My entire life can be described in one sentence:
It didn't go as planned, and that's OK."

— Rachel Wolchin

- As we've discussed, chronic illness is a significant form of loss. And one of our needs in trying to integrate the loss and the ongoing reality of the illness into our lives is to tell the story.

- Telling the story of our illness helps it hold together. When we tell someone else the story of how we became sick, the steps and trials we went through during diagnosis, and the symptoms, treatment, and life journey we've been on ever since, we are creating a narrative. We are making all the chaotic days and incidents cohere to form a true-life story.

- Stories help us make sense of the world and ourselves. They also help others understand what we are going through.

- So don't be afraid to tell your story. Tell others when it comes up or when you feel compelled. Write your story in a journal or on a blog. Paint your story on a canvas. Live your story by serving others with similar needs. No matter how you tell your story, the telling of it will help you live a fuller and more genuine and connected life.

- Do keep in mind, you can usually tell that some people want to hold up your story, while others don't. It's OK to be selective with when, where, and with whom you feel safe to share your story.

CARPE DIEM
Tell at least part of your story in some way today.

16.

PRIORITIZE REST AND SLEEP

"Resting is not laziness, it's medicine!"

— Glenn Schweitzer

- Those of us with chronic illness may have several daily, can't-miss self-care regimens.

- Medication? Check. Testing? Check. Treatment? Check.

- It's important to remember that good-quality rest and sleep are also critical to our health.

- Simply put, our bodies may need good rest and sleep more than most because our conditions sap our energy and require regular time for recuperation and repair. When you're tired, rest. Better yet, learn to rest yourself regularly *before* you get overtired.

- Are your rest and sleep habits serving you well? If not, talk to your primary-care provider about your challenges. Insomnia, sleep apnea, restless-leg syndrome, frequent waking, light sleeping, chronic fatigue, and other issues will almost certainly exacerbate your chronic illness and severely compromise your quality of life. Don't let sleep issues go on and on. Take action.

CARPE DIEM
Take action to prioritize good-quality rest and sleep today.

17.

LISTEN TO YOUR BODY—AND SOUL

"Self-care has become a new priority—the revelation that it's perfectly permissible to listen to your body and do what it needs."

— Frances Ryan

- Most of us are good at paying attention to our thoughts. Our minds like to run the show. In fact, it's easy to slip into the misconception that we *are* our minds.

- For many of us, learning to listen to our bodies often takes conscious practice. Right now, close your eyes and mentally scan your body, starting at the toes and working upward. What is your body feeling? Does it hurt anywhere? Is there good energy or a desire to move anywhere? It is cold? Hot? Comfortable? Full? Empty? Tired?

- When we become more attuned to our bodies, we get better at taking care of them and treating them as they need to be treated.

- Learning to listen to our souls can also be challenging but offers great reward. When we meditate, pray, spend time in nature, and engage in other spiritual practices, we connect to and feed our souls. We discover our divine sparks—that timeless flicker within us that yearns for meaning and purpose.

- The more we learn to turn off our minds and listen, the better our lives will be.

CARPE DIEM
Set aside two 15-minute time-outs today.
Spend the first listening to and taking care of your body.
Spend the second listening to and taking care of your soul.

18.

REMEMBER SELF-RESPECT

"Love yourself first, and everything else falls into line.
You really have to love yourself to get anything done in this world."

— Lucille Ball

- Self-respect is essential to wellbeing for everyone. The capacity for excellent self-care and self-compassion—not to mention self-fulfillment—comes from a strong foundation of self-respect.

- When those of us with chronic illness live from a foundation of self-respect, not only are we kind to ourselves and take good care of ourselves, we also consistently strive to live our best lives—and forgive ourselves when we make choices that take us on less healthy paths.

- Self-respect is also about congruency (see Idea 49) and honest, kind communication, with ourselves and with others.

- For many people with chronic illness, another thing self-respect demands is not giving in to the temptation of thinking of ourselves as victims or "less than." Yes, we live with physical or mental-health issues. But almost everyone lives with challenges of some kind—challenges that may not be apparent to the world.

- Self-love and self-respect are at the heart of this book. Everything builds from there.

CARPE DIEM
Is there some way in which you haven't been respecting yourself?
Address it today.

19.

PUT YOURSELF FIRST

*"Most of the shadows in this life are caused by
standing in one's own sunshine."*
— Ralph Waldo Emerson

- Before helping others, put your own oxygen mask on first. If you've flown much, you've heard this instruction umpteen times.

- It's good advice. After all, you won't be able to help people who are dependent on you if you're not functional yourself.

- This same strategy applies to chronic illness. If you don't take good care of yourself, not only will your health and quality of life suffer, you won't be in a position to support the people you love, either. And they'll be further hurt watching you suffer or go downhill.

- So give yourself permission to put yourself first. It's what's best for you, and it's also what's best for all the important people in your life. It's truly a win-win scenario.

CARPE DIEM

If you're not used to putting yourself first, it can feel awkward or selfish
at first. In some way, prioritize your own needs today. Keep doing
it until it becomes second nature and the awkwardness fades.

20.

IDENTIFY YOUR HELPERS

*"One who knows how to show and to accept kindness will be
a friend better than any possession."*
— Sophocles

- When it comes to chronic illness, not everyone is equipped to be a helper. And some people are good at helping with some aspects of the challenge but not other aspects.

- First, it's important that we acknowledge that some people don't have the capacity to be a helper. That doesn't mean they're bad people; it just means they have other strengths and styles.

- Some of the people who are not naturally good helpers are likely among those closest to us—our friends and family members. We can't change them, but we can try to appreciate them for who they are, just as we want them to appreciate us for who we are.

- I (Alan) often talk about the "rule of thirds." In my experience, about one third of people in your life are neutral when it comes to dealing with your challenging needs. They don't help you or hurt you. One third can be toxic and may end up making you feel worse than you did before you were in their presence. And one third will be your empathetic, hope-filled companions.

- Whenever you need help and support, identify and seek out your friends and family who are in the last group. They will be your rocks. Some among the first group may be good at helping with practical tasks or just having fun with. Avoid the second group, especially when you're feeling vulnerable. And try to understand that their shortcomings are actually about deep-seated pain in their own lives—not about you.

CARPE DIEM
Who is in your helpers group? Thank them in some way today.

21.

PRACTICE INTENTION-SETTING

"You either get bitter or you get better. It's that simple. You either take what has been dealt to you and allow it to make you a better person, or you allow it to tear you down. The choice does not belong to fate, it belongs to you."
— Josh Shipp

- Intention-setting is a self-care practice that guides us to be aware of what we desire and to articulate that desire so that we can make micro-decisions moment-by-moment to achieve it. A close cousin to "affirmation," it is using the power of clarity of thought to steer ourselves toward a desired result.

- When you set your intention to manage your chronic illness or proceed through the day in a certain way, you make a true commitment to positively influence the course of your journey. You choose between being a "passive witness" or an "active participant" in your experience.

- The concept of intention-setting presupposes that your outer reality is in part a reflection of your inner thoughts and beliefs. If you can change or mold some of your thoughts and beliefs, then you can influence your reality. And in journaling and speaking (and praying!) your intentions, you help "set" them.

- Try setting your intention for the day at the beginning of each morning. It can be something as simple as "I intend to practice patience today" or "Today I will smile at each person I interact with," or it could be something grander, such as "I am filled with hope and healing." At the end of the day, journal about what your intention for the day accomplished and consider tomorrow's intention.

CARPE DIEM
Set your intention for this day or, if it's already late in the day, for tomorrow.

22.

KEEP A JOURNAL

"Health is a journal your body keeps about you."
— Terri Guillemets

- Before you skip this idea because you're not a writer, please indulge us for a moment. Because keeping a journal isn't just for writers.

- Journaling is an effective way of getting your thoughts and feelings outside yourself. It's not about the words or the quality of the writing itself; it's about expression and unburdening.

- Journaling can help you whenever you're feeling anxious, upset, angry, sad, guilty, or any other challenging feeling. Just spend a few minutes putting those feelings on paper and *voila!*—notice how much better you feel.

- Your journal can have a wide or narrow focus. You may choose to make daily notes about your chronic-illness symptoms and what is helping you feel better (or worse). Or you might keep a hope journal, in which you write down your hopes and dreams about the future. Or you could just make simple lists of impressions from your day—maybe things that made you smile.

- You don't have to be a master chef to prepare a healthy, delicious meal, and you don't have to be a writer to keep a journal. You just have to be willing to give it a try.

CARPE DIEM
Try journaling for five minutes today.

23.

BE AWARE OF DENIAL

"Denial is a useful defense mechanism until it's not."
— Rosalind Kaplan

- When something bad happens to us, denial can be a wonderful tool—in the short term. It helps us survive traumatic moments that would otherwise be unsurvivable. Shock, numbness, and denial are nature's gift to us in the immediate aftermath of bad news or a terrible experience. They are like bubble wrap protecting our hearts and souls.

- Many of us have experienced shock, numbness, and denial at various points in our chronic-illness journeys. We may have felt shocked and numb after hearing the news of our diagnosis. We might have been in denial sometimes about our need to take medication or monitor our health closely.

- While shock, numbness, and denial have protective qualities in the short term, they are counterproductive in the long term. To deny that we are ill and need special care is to deny ourselves the best health we can achieve and maintain. Denial of our unique needs and possible limitations undermines our ability to live our best lives.

- Being fully open to, conscious of, and attentive to our reality, on the other hand, allows us to live our truths and receive the care and support we need. The opposite of denial is acknowledgment. Attuning to and fully acknowledging our changing circumstances each day is not only responsible, it's life-affirming.

CARPE DIEM

Are you stuck in shock, numbness, or denial about any aspect of your chronic illness? If so, take one small step today to break through.

24.

ESTABLISH SPIRITUAL PRACTICES THAT WORK FOR YOU

"With spiritual balance...you are able to deal with whatever life brings you and know you are OK. You are able to find meaning and purpose even in situations that are painful and not to your liking."

— Dr. Mel Pohl

- Loss, grief, and mourning are first and foremost spiritual journeys. Yes, they affect us physically, cognitively, emotionally, and socially, too, but because they stem from our deepest desires, hopes, and loves, they are the biggest and most profound challenges we will face in our lifetime.

- Spiritual challenges are most effectively met with spiritual practices.

- Whether you ascribe to a religion, to spiritual beliefs, or simply to spiritual skepticism or seeking, spiritual practices will help you explore your spirituality and your ideas about meaning and purpose in this life and beyond.

- We recommend setting aside half an hour for spirit each day. You can use this time for any practices that help you feel more in tune with your inner spark, nature, God, and the universe. Meditation, prayer, walks in nature, yoga, expressing gratitude, creating artwork, offering service to others, and many other activities can help you feed your soul and move deeper into a life of meaning and purpose.

CARPE DIEM
Set aside half an hour for spiritual practice today. Spend the time on a spiritual activity you already know works for you, or try something new.

25.

REALIZE THAT BEING VULNERABLE IS BEING STRONG

"Daring greatly means the courage to be vulnerable. It means to show up and be seen. To ask for what you need. To talk about how you're feeling. To have the hard conversations."

— Dr. Brené Brown

- Some chronically ill people have a tendency to keep a stiff upper lip. They don't want to complain, inconvenience others, or "bore" people with the details of their treatment and prognosis, so they wear the armor of "I'm fine" and "Don't worry about me" and "Nothing to see here." Does any of that sound familiar?

- But the paradox is, it actually takes more courage to be vulnerable. It's scarier to zip open our chests and let others see our griefs, our fears, and even our most cherished hopes.

- Dare to be vulnerable. If you're not used to or good at it yet, start small. Tell one person one minor but meaningful truth about yourself that you don't usually talk about. See what happens.

- Explaining your illness to others may seem hard. You may think they can't truly understand. But those who care about you want to listen. Being surrounded by people who know what you're experiencing can make the sometimes hidden world of chronic illness feel seen and help you feel more whole and truly you.

- When you allow yourself to become more and more vulnerable, what you are really opening yourself to is more life—more potential pain, yes, but also more meaning and joy. What you'll find is that the hurt that sometimes comes with vulnerability is well worth the profound gifts of presence, truth, and connection.

CARPE DIEM
Make yourself vulnerable in some small but meaningful way today.

26.

MEDITATE

*"Meditation is a vital way to purify and quiet the mind,
thus rejuvenating the body."*
— Deepak Chopra

- Daily meditation can help us in many ways. It can help us connect to and strengthen our divine sparks. It can help us feel less cognitively stressed. And it can even ease our experience of our physical symptoms.

- Really? Meditation can help our bodies? It can. Our physical symptoms of chronic illness, which for some people includes chronic pain, are often exacerbated by our emotions about those symptoms as well as by the stories we tell ourselves about those symptoms. Meditation can soften our negative emotions and help us create more affirming stories.

- When you experience an unwanted physical symptom of your illness, do you get upset, angry, or annoyed? If so, those feelings, while natural and understandable, are likely worsening your physical symptom. That's because when we're upset, our bodies release stress chemicals and activate inflammatory responses. If we use meditation to observe and accept our challenging emotions, instead, those feelings attenuate, and so our physical symptoms may also attenuate.

- The stories we tell ourselves about our physical symptoms also play a role. Old saws like, "I'm always sick," "Life's not fair," and "I'm never going to feel better" only serve to compound the body's stress reaction. It's a vicious cycle. Through meditation, we can choose to replace those self-damaging stories with others that serve us better. Meditating on life-affirming mantras such as, "I am grateful for this day," "I am enough," and "My intention today is _____," has the power to transform our life experience.

CARPE DIEM
Meditate today using the life-affirming mantra you most need right now.

27.

LIVE IN THE NOW

"And here you are living, despite it all."
— Rupi Kaur

- Have you ever had the privilege of knowing someone with a disability or chronic disease who seemed to exude nothing but hope, joy, and kindness?

- That's what living in the now can do for us. It orients us to squeeze as much life out of every moment as we can to the extent that we can.

- Of course, sometimes living in the now with chronic illness means experiencing and addressing our symptoms. When we are tired, we should rest. When we are grieving, we mourn. When we are hurting, we turn to the healthy pain-control methods that work for us. There is also meaning in taking care of ourselves.

- The amazing thing about living in the now is that there are miracles in every moment. Right now, look around you—even if you're in bed! Turn on your five senses. What can you see, touch, taste, smell, and hear that is worthy of wonder and gratitude?

- Living in the now is about not focusing on what we're missing out on but rather focusing on what we're present for. The grass is always greener on the other side, the saying goes, but the truth is that the greenest grass is always the grass where your toes are planted.

CARPE DIEM

Look around you right now and get in touch with all five of your senses. What do you see? Smell? Hear? Taste? Feel? Home in on one of the senses and sit in wonder and appreciation of it for a minute or two.

28.

MAKE THE MOST OF MEDICAL VISITS

"Physicians and patients need to work together to pursue care that improves health, avoids harms, and eliminates wasteful practices."

— Dr. Amir Qaseem

- Those of us who are chronically ill often have a love-hate relationship with our healthcare providers. We love them for helping us manage our symptoms and the course of our illness. And we hate them for all the poking, prodding, naysaying, medicating, and time-taking they have to do.

- Basically, being chronically ill can seem like an unwanted full-time job—in addition to being an unwanted full-time state of being.

- But if we change our thinking about our medical visits, we can reshape the experience. First, we can create a brief, efficient ritual of preparation for each visit. Perhaps we spend five minutes the night or morning before thinking through the purpose of the visit and jotting down any questions we want to be sure to ask. Keeping a medical notebook helps with this. Second, we can make sure we're being team players. It's not us versus our care providers. It's us as lead team member. And third, we can work to have gratitude for every poke and prod. No, the system isn't perfect, but we are fortunate to live in a time when healthcare is better than it has ever been. Thank goodness for doctors and nurses. Thank goodness for holistic providers. Thank goodness for imaging technology, surgical developments, treatment improvements, effective medication, kind words, and smiles.

- Healthcare may be a right, but it's also a privilege. Let's make the most of it.

CARPE DIEM
Today, prepare for your next medical visit by making some notes and setting reminders.

29.

IF YOU'RE IN PAIN, SEEK HELP

"Time is not a cure for chronic pain, but it can be crucial for improvement. It takes time to change, to recover, and to make progress."
— Dr. Mel Pohl

• Chronic pain is without a doubt one of the most challenging and prevalent aspects of chronic illness. According to the Centers for Disease Control, 50 million Americans live with chronic pain. About 20 million of them have what is termed "high-impact chronic pain," meaning it's severe enough that it often limits their life or work.

• If you're among those experiencing chronic pain, we're sorry—and we're aware that there is often not a simple solution. It's outside the scope of this book to review chronic-pain treatment options, but know that there are a number of avenues and resources available, from physical therapy and pain medication to acupuncture, massage, meditation, exercise, nerve stimulation, psychological therapies, and more.

• Pain-specialist physicians emphasize that people should not have to live with chronic pain. Many believe that an individualized combination of options can be crafted to help every person.

• If you have not yet found pain-relief therapies that work for you, please keep trying. Seek a second or third opinion from different pain specialists. Get advice from others who've found paths through chronic pain. Be as tenacious as your pain, and give yourself permission to be needy of ample love, support, and self-compassion.

CARPE DIEM
If you're in pain, seek help today.

30.

IF YOU'RE YOUNG, ESTABLISH GOOD HABITS EARLY

"Good habits formed at youth make all the difference."
— Aristotle

- Chronic illness is not a sprint, it's a marathon. In fact, it's often a lifelong marathon.

- The sooner we establish good daily habits, the better our quality of life will be in both the short term and the long run. It's as simple as that.

- Good physical self-care is one essential array of habits. But taking care of ourselves cognitively, emotionally, socially, and spiritually on a daily basis is also necessary.

- The thing about good habits is that they don't really take that much extra time or energy. Yet when you add them all up, they make a world of difference in how we feel and experience our lives.

- And if you're not young? As the saying goes, the best time to plant a tree is 20 years ago. The second best time to plant a tree is right now.

CARPE DIEM
Educate yourself about the best daily habits that someone with your condition should strive for. Start working on them today.

31.

REFRAME THE CONCEPT OF "BATTLING" TO SUIT YOU

"It's not the situation that's causing your stress, it's your thoughts, and you can change that right here and now. You can choose to be peaceful right here and now. Peace is a choice, and it has nothing to do with what other people do or think."
— Gerald G. Jampolsky, M.D.

- The idea of "battling illness" has been prominent in our culture's thinking for centuries. We talk of people fighting valiantly or courageously against cancer and other life-threatening diseases. And when they die, we also sometimes say that they lost their battle.

- The war metaphor of disease makes sense and feels motivating to some people. To others it feels inaccurate, hollow, or even blameful. After all, if you are fighting an illness but despite your best efforts it gets the better of you, you might feel that you didn't fight hard or well enough, right? Some studies have shown that people who view their disease as an "enemy" tend to have higher levels of depression and anxiety as well as worse quality of life.

- Each of us experiencing chronic illness gets to decide. Are we battling our disease, or are we befriending it? Are we waging war, or we making peace? Are we eradicating, or are we controlling or managing?

- There's no right answer. There's only what works for you and serves as a tool for helping you live your best life. Just know that it's a choice. *Your* choice.

CARPE DIEM
Spend a few minutes considering how you feel about the idea of "battling" your illness. If you'd like, you can decide to reorient your thinking and the words you use.

32.

EXAMINE YOUR BELIEFS
ABOUT BEING SICK

*"I fight for my health every day in ways that most people
don't understand. I'm not lazy. I'm a warrior!"*

— Unknown

- When we're children, we learn many values and ways of being from our parents and other influential grown-ups. Some of these lessons are explicitly stated, while others are unspoken rules and judgments.

- Think for a few minutes about the values, rules, and judgments about illness that were dominant in your family. What did you learn or absorb about how sickness should be thought of and how sick people should be treated?

- Was illness considered a weakness, or was it indulged? Did people feign or exaggerate sickness in order to be taken care of by others? Were doctors treated with deference? Or were doctor visits rare because they were too costly or "unnecessary"? Was illness spoken about openly and honestly, or was it hidden or shameful? Was the science of illness and treatment respected or ignored?

- Now consider how those values, rules, and judgments shape, still to this day, your experience of your own chronic illness. Do they help or hinder you?

- Examining your beliefs about illness can help you understand them— and modify them if you want to. You have the power to choose only beliefs that make you feel understood, supported, and loved. No, you can't change what others believe, but you can change your own self-talk so that it's supportive and loving.

CARPE DIEM
Spend a few minutes today talking to someone else about your
beliefs and theirs surrounding sickness. Compare notes.
Consider how those beliefs serve you today.

33.

CRY WHEN YOU FEEL LIKE CRYING

*"There must be those among whom we can sit down
and weep and still be counted as warriors."*

— Adrienne Rich

- Crying is such an effective way to express our grief—in other words, to mourn. It's our body's natural mechanism for expressing itself during times of acute distress and ridding itself of stress hormones.

- Did you know there are three different types of human tears, each with their own chemical make-up? Basal tears keep our eyes lubricated, reflex tears wash harmful gases away (such as when we chop onions), and psychic tears release strong emotions such as happiness and sadness.

- So when you feel like crying, cry! It's good for your body, and it's good for your heart and soul. It's taking the feelings you have on the inside and expressing them on the outside, which is so important in living with chronic-illness grief.

- Not everyone is a crier, so if you rarely feel like crying, that's OK too. You still feel emotions, though, so it's nonetheless essential to learn to pay attention to them and express them in ways that suit you.

CARPE DIEM
The next time you feel like crying, allow yourself to cry.
Notice how you feel afterward.

34.

PRACTICE EQUANIMITY

*"Deep down, nature is inherently peaceful, calm, and beautiful.
The universe as a whole is perfect. The chaos is on the surface."*

— Amit Ray

- Equanimity means maintaining inner and outer calm and composure even in the midst of chaos or strife. Think level-headedness, self-possession, Zen.

- With chronic illness, we often can't fully control what happens to us or what happens around us. But we can learn to respond mindfully and calmly to challenging circumstances.

- The benefits of cultivated equanimity are many, including lower levels of harmful stress hormones in our bodies, a calmer presence and experience of the world, wiser reactions when a truly time-sensitive crisis arises, and kinder treatment of others, to name just a few.

- Meditation, yoga, biofeedback, cognitive behavioral therapy, and other mindfulness tools can teach us how to respond and live with equanimity. Anyone can do it; it just takes practice.

CARPE DIEM
Today, when something doesn't go your way, try responding
with intentional equanimity. Use mindful breathing (Idea 5)
in the heat of the moment if you need support.
Notice how you feel after practicing equanimity.

35.

UNDERSTAND THE MIND-BODY CONNECTION

*"Your health is what you make of it.
Everything you do and think either adds to the vitality,
energy, and spirit you possess or takes away from it."*
— Ann Wigmore

- Our bodies respond to our thoughts and emotions. Patterns of anxious or negative thoughts and emotions can make our chronic illnesses worse.

- Our bodies operate via biochemistry. Neurological pathways connect our brains with our muscles and organs. When we think distressing thoughts or feel distressing emotions, our brains direct the release of hormones and neurotransmitters to all our bodily systems, communicating a biochemical SOS and suppressing our immune systems. Did you know, for example, that studies have shown that cancer patients whose depression was eased through group therapy went on to live longer?

- Mindfulness practices like meditation, yoga, hypnotherapy, tai chi, and others not only help us experience more peace and calm, they may well also lessen our chronic-illness symptoms.

- Simply put, our lives get better when we learn to appreciate and harness the mind-body connection.

CARPE DIEM
Spend half an hour on a mindfulness practice of your choosing today.

36.

UNDERSTAND THE DIFFERENCE BETWEEN ISOLATION AND SOLITUDE

"Loneliness expresses the pain of being alone,
and solitude expresses the glory of being alone."
— Paul Tillich

- When we are feeling the pain—physical or emotional—of our chronic illness, we may naturally withdraw. It's normal to seek shelter from the outside world in such moments.

- In addition to physical respite, we need the stillness of alone time to feel our feelings and think our thoughts. To slow down and to turn inward, we must sometimes cultivate solitude. Being alone is not the curse some people make it out to be. It is actually a blessing. After all, we are born alone, and we will die alone. We are each by ourselves a child of the universe.

- But sometimes those of us who are chronically ill self-isolate too much. We cut ourselves off from others because it seems easier or more practical. Solitude is productive, but isolation is reductive. As with so many things in life, it's a question of balance and proportion.

- If we are overdoing isolation, we must find ways to reach out to others. We can establish new routines of spending time with friends, family members, neighbors, work colleagues, likeminded hobbyists, and others with whom we have things in common. Not only does working on connection enrich our lives in general, it provides us with a support network for times when we need practical help or are in despair.

CARPE DIEM

Take a moment to assess your solitude vs. isolation balance. How do you think you're doing? Which do you need more or less of? Do a reality check by asking a good friend how they think you're doing in this area.

37.

FIND OTHERS WHO "GET IT"

"Do not believe the things you tell yourself when you're sad and alone."
— Unknown

- You're on a unique, personal journey, but you're not alone. Others are also living with the same or similar chronic illness. No two people will have the exact same experience, but there's enough overlap and commonalities that it's almost always more than worthwhile to seek out "your people." Finding others with the same illness can make you feel truly understood and help you lend a hand to others who are going through the same struggles and frustrations you are.

- Online forums are a convenient way to communicate with other people who share your experience. One of the great things about online groups and social- media forums is that you can share as much or as little as you'd like, but you can read all you want. The feeling of connection builds quickly, and people are often highly supportive of one another as well as forthcoming about things like symptom relief, treatment successes, and more.

- Face-to-face support groups are another good option, especially for more common chronic illnesses. Ask your specialist about support groups in the community, or call your local hospital or library to find area options.

- We hope you have some friends and family members who are strong supporters and good listeners. But even if you do, participating in a community of people who share your experience and "get it" will meet needs that your friends and family cannot.

CARPE DIEM
Reach out today to establish and strengthen a connection
with someone who "gets it."

38.

REPURPOSE EMBARRASSMENT

---

*"Promise me you'll always remember: You're braver than you believe,
and stronger than you seem, and smarter than you think."*

— A. A. Milne

- Those of us with chronic illness know that sometimes, no matter how much we plan and prepare, our bodies can do embarrassing things.

- Depending on which chronic illness we're living with, on any given day we might seize, fall, panic, faint, soil ourselves, or experience any number of public—and sometimes dangerous—humiliations.

- To avoid such embarrassments, it can be tempting to just stay home all the time. But unless we're truly homebound by our illnesses, choosing isolation over participation only limits our lives.

- Instead, we can choose to repurpose embarrassment. We can use such moments to put on our teaching hats and educate others about what happened and why. Or we can emphasize the absurdity of being human and tell a joke. Or we can leverage the intimacy with others these situations often give rise to. Maybe we can even take the opportunity to make a new friend or grow closer to an existing companion.

- It's normal and natural to feel embarrassed when our bodies betray us, but remember what we said about vulnerability (Idea 25): it opens us to the gifts of presence, truth, and connection.

CARPE DIEM
Think about a way in which your chronic illness sometimes embarrasses you. Now think about how you can reframe this situation as an opportunity.

39.

SPARK HOPE

"When the unthinkable happens, the lighthouse is hope.
Once we choose hope, everything is possible."
— Christopher Reeve

- Hope is an expectation of a good that is yet to be. It is forward-looking, but we feel it buoy us in the now.

- Hope is so essential to living well with chronic illness that we think fostering it should belong on every reader's daily to-do list.

- So how do we spark hope? First, by recognizing and acknowledging it when we feel it, and second, by intentionally devoting time to it each and every day.

- First, think about what makes you feel hopeful. Brainstorm a written list if you want. Anything that makes you feel that bright spark of hope about tomorrow, next week, next month, next year, or even years from now belongs on the list. Your hope-sparkers can be both little things (such as a coming gathering with friends) and big things (such as the goal of buying a house or taking a trip).

- Second, think about ways you could integrate hope into every day. Here are some ideas: Make plans to see a friend you haven't seen in a while. Meditate on a message of hope. Make reservations at a favorite restaurant. Put a book, audiobook, or film you're excited about on hold at the library. Read hopeful articles and stories about others living well with a chronic condition. Schedule a vacation or staycation. Spend five minutes each day visualizing your desired future. Create a vision board.

- Our illnesses are not a choice, but hope is a choice. Let's choose it.

CARPE DIEM
Intentionally integrate hope into this day. Repeat tomorrow
and tomorrow and tomorrow, ad infinitum.

40.

LOOK FOR FINANCIAL HELP

"The strong individual is the one who asks for help when he needs it."
— Rona Barrett

- If healthcare costs, work limitations, childcare expenses, or other monetary demands related to your chronic illness have put you or your family in a financial bind, it's part of your commitment to excellent self-care to look into options for financial help.

- A number of patient-assistance programs help pay for or reduce the cost of prescription drugs. Google "prescription drug assistance."

- Local nonprofits such as faith communities and United Way agencies often provide no-strings-attached emergency grants to help pay for food, housing, medical expenses, and more. Call your local United Way, or visit 211.org.

- You may qualify for government assistance, such as reduced housing costs, food benefits, or Medicaid. Consider it essential self-care to apply for such help when you need it.

- Caring Voice Coalition is a nonprofit dedicated to helping people with chronic illness. Visit caringvoice.org.

CARPE DIEM
If you need financial help, look into options today. Brainstorm with a compassionate friend or family member if it helps you to talk things out.

41.

FORGE INTIMATE RELATIONSHIPS

"Souls tend to go back to who feels like home."
— N.R. Heart

- We've already talked about the importance of reaching out to others for love and support as well as socializing. It's not debatable: For most of us, love and human connection are paramount to living well.

- Intimate relationships are those in which we share our most tender, vulnerable selves with another human being. Such relationships may or may not be sexual. We can have soulmate relationships with best friends and family members too. (And sexual relationships are not necessarily intimate; intimacy requires emotional bonding as well.)

- Chronic illness can sometimes seem like a barrier to intimate relationships. We have this "problem" that we don't want to burden others with, or that we presume is off-putting to others, so we may avoid getting too close to anyone.

- We must love ourselves enough to realize that we, too, need and deserve loving, intimate relationships. Chances are that those with whom we would form intimate bonds also have challenges of their own. We are enough. And someone else will be as lucky to have us as we will be to have them.

CARPE DIEM
Nurture an intimate relationship today.

42.

CREATE PREDICTABILITY

"My own prescription for health is less paperwork and more running barefoot through the grass."
— Terri Guillemets

- Part of what can be so exhausting about living with chronic illness is, at least for some of us, the daily, constant uncertainty. Will we be able to do something planned or won't we? Will we feel OK or won't we? Will our bodies hold up that day or won't they?

- Creating and living with healthy routines can help give our days structure and predictability despite the uncertainty about how we'll feel or how our bodies may respond. If we always get up at a certain time followed by a period of meditation, making our beds, a healthy breakfast, and a short walk, we can take comfort and find solidity in this routine.

- Other elements of positive predictability we can install in our lives might include caring for a pet or plants, scheduling regular contact with friends and family, and engaging in regular recreational activities that give us joy.

- If, on the other hand, predictability in your life has turned into boredom, the opposite is called for. If you're bored with your daily routines, try creating unpredictability instead. Work to add something new, slightly scary, or fresh. Just one simple burst of novelty each day—a food, a TV show, a place, an article of clothing—can be enough to reengage your spirit.

CARPE DIEM
Rethink your morning routine for tomorrow.
If you need more healthy predictability, commit to that.
If you need something fresh, add novelty.

43.

JOIN OR CREATE A SUPPORT GROUP

"The best thing to hold onto in life is each other."
— Audrey Hepburn

• Living with a chronic illness gets easier when we have the ongoing support of others. When some of those others know just what it's like to live with the same chronic illness? Even better.

• Participating in a support group gives us the gift of true understanding. It helps us feel we are not alone. In fact, our support-group friendships can develop over time into one of the pillars of our lives.

• Look for chronic-illness support groups in your community. If you can't find something suitable locally, you may be able to find an exact match for your illness online. And it's not either-or. You can join a local support group *and* an online community.

• If you can't find a support group that's a good fit, maybe you can create one. Talk to your healthcare providers, friends, and family about assembling a group of three or four people with chronic illness to meet and share stories. You might be surprised by the level of interest.

CARPE DIEM
Look into support groups today.

44.

LOOK FOR THE HUMOR

*"A good laugh and a long sleep are the
best cures in the doctor's book."*

— Irish proverb

- Some of the things we have to deal with as part of our chronic
  illness are simply absurd.

- Have you ever found yourself shaking your head in disbelief or
  chuckling at the absurdity of a symptom, outcome, or circumstance?

- Human existence in a human body can be ridiculous, that's for sure.
  Sometimes we may want to cry, but sometimes we feel like laughing.

- We can learn to cultivate our senses of humor when it comes to the
  vagaries of our chronic illnesses. Instead of living in fear, anxiety,
  disappointment, anger, or sadness all the time, we can learn to laugh
  things off sometimes.

- By now you know that we (Alan and Jaimie) would never advocate
  denying natural grief and faking happiness instead. That's not what
  we mean here. What we mean is that even as we embrace challenging
  thoughts and feelings, we can still choose to laugh and appreciate the
  absurd.

CARPE DIEM
Who do you know who has a good sense of humor?
Talk to that person today. Ask them how they laugh off
challenging moments in their life.

45.

MANAGE EXPECTATIONS

"My happiness grows in direct proportion to my acceptance, and in inverse proportion to my expectations."

— Michael J. Fox

- One way to define contentment is the matching of our expectations with reality. When we expect something to be a certain way and it is, we often find ourselves content. We may not be thrilled, but on the other hand, we may not be disappointed, either.

- Because we must live with a chronic illness, learning to manage our expectations can help us find more contentment and equilibrium in our days.

- Things don't always have to be wonderful or above-average to be meaningful. We can find joy and meaning in ordinary moments if we simply reframe our thinking. This, in fact, is the goal of mindfulness practices.

- And when we manage our expectations so that we're able to achieve contentment and find meaning no matter what happens, sometimes we'll be happily surprised. Now and then something will occur that will exceed our managed expectations. How delicious is our delight in those moments.

CARPE DIEM

Consider your expectations for something on your schedule today or tomorrow. How could you reframe or rescale those expectations to find meaning and joy in whatever happens?

46.

EXAMINE THE FLIP SIDE

"Too many people miss the silver lining because they're expecting gold."
— Maurice Setter

- Whenever things don't go our way, it's natural to get frustrated and feel angry, sad, or any number of challenging feelings. Those feelings are part of our normal loss and grief journey.

- Acknowledging and befriending our feelings—*all* our feelings, even the "bad" ones—as they arise is an essential habit to cultivate as we strive to live our best lives.

- At the same time we're working on this type of self-awareness and self-compassion, we're also working on creating a holding place for hope and joy. With intention, we're both befriending our grief *and* actively seeking happiness and meaning.

- So whenever things don't go our way, we can also look on the flip side. Has the unwanted fork in the road also created any new, potentially positive opportunities? Are there any silver linings? The answer is almost always "yes."

- Looking at both the dark and the bright sides at the same time isn't denial—it's holistic, authentic, hopeful awareness.

CARPE DIEM
When something bad or challenging happens today, stop to consider the flip side.

47.

SPEND YOUR ENERGY BUDGET INTENTIONALLY

"Energy is the essence of life. Every day you decide how you're going to use it by knowing what you want and what it takes to reach that goal, and by maintaining focus."
— Oprah Winfrey

- Our energy is a limited resource. That's true of everyone, but especially those of us with chronic illness.

- Think of your energy as a daily budget. You have X hours of physical stamina, X hours of mental focus, and X hours of emotional/spiritual energy to spend each day. Once your budget is spent, you need to rest and recharge for tomorrow.

- How will you spend today's budget? Make a list of your most important to-do items and match them up with your available hours of energy. Also align times of day that you feel most energetic with the tasks that require the most energy.

- Be intentional. You can choose to allocate energy only to tasks that are necessary or that you really care about. Don't waste your precious limited resources on time-wasters that don't matter to you.

- Don't forget to budget some cream-of-the-crop energy each day for baby steps toward your bucket-list hopes, dreams, and goals. A year from now, what will you be sad about not having done if you don't do it? Whatever that desire is, it deserves some of your best energy today, tomorrow, and the next day.

CARPE DIEM
Create your energy-budget plan for tomorrow.

48.

TRY OUT DIFFERENT RESPONSES TO "THE QUESTION"

"I realized there is no shame in being honest.
There is no shame in being vulnerable. It's the beauty of being human."
— Unknown

- How are you? The answer to this simple question isn't simple at all for many people with chronic illness.

- On the one hand, we're thankful people ask. On the other hand, we don't believe they really, actually, truly want the true or full story in response.

- We (Alan and Jaimie) believe that honesty and vulnerability serve both you and the asker best. But conciseness is also a good idea. So try being truthful and brief. For example, you might say something like, "I've been having some trouble with seizures lately, but I'm on a new medication that seems promising. I appreciate you asking. How are you?"

- Try out different responses until you find a few that work for you. Keep in mind that the pat response "I'm fine" doesn't build bonds or understanding. Instead, it's a kind of wall that keeps the truth at bay. Genuine connection only happens through genuine communication. Dare to be honest. Dare to be you.

CARPE DIEM
The next time you're asked, "How are you?—try a new response.
Be genuine, honest, and brief. Notice what happens.

49.

BE HONEST—WITH YOURSELF AND WITH OTHERS

"Real transformation requires real honesty.
If you want to move forward, get real with yourself."
— Bryant McGill

- In psychology, there's a concept called "congruency" that is pertinent to living our best lives with chronic illness.

- Basically, congruency means living in ways consistent with our internal beliefs, values, and true feelings. For example, if we value kindness and we treat others with kindness, we are living congruently. If, however, we value kindness but are unkind to others, we are living incongruently.

- Incongruency is being dishonest with ourselves. Incongruency injures our hearts and souls. Conversely, congruency enriches our lives and multiplies our feelings of meaning and purpose. Congruency is essential to being our best selves.

- Of course, incongruency is also being dishonest with others. When we hide or misrepresent our true beliefs, values, and feelings, we're lying to the world, including the people we care about.

- It's true what you've heard about truth—it sets us free.

CARPE DIEM
Identify one way in which you are living incongruently.
Today, talk about it with someone else, or take action to address it.

50.

DEVELOP SKILLS FOR DEALING WITH WORRY

"You can't calm the storm, so stop trying.
What you can do is calm yourself. The storm will pass."
— Timber Hawkeye

- It's normal to experience anxiety. Living with a chronic illness sometimes means worrying about upcoming test results, worsening symptoms, life situations or expectations made more challenging by the illness, financial issues, and more.

- To some degree, this kind of anxiety is helpful because it spurs us to complete essential tasks: to visit the doctor, make plans to accommodate challenging situations, seek financial support, etc. In other words, anxiety is often the kick in the pants we need to take proactive action.

- But ongoing, daily, unacted-upon anxiety is unhelpful. Stress hormones can make us more sick. And constant worry constantly ruins our experience of the present.

- Self-help books, videos, counselors, and mindfulness practices can all help us develop skills for proactively and positively managing anxiety. If you're often anxious, working to build a menu of anxiety-management skills that work for you must become an essential part of your self-care regimen.

CARPE DIEM
Today, take one concrete step toward developing a new
anxiety-management skill. Take another step tomorrow.

51.

PRACTICE HOPEFUL SELF-TALK

"Talk to yourself like you would to someone you love."
— Dr. Brené Brown

- How we talk to ourselves in the privacy of our minds has a toxic effect on our quality of life.

- We know from numerous psychology studies that human beings are prone to negative self-talk, which has, as you might guess, negative effects.

- Negative self-talk results in higher stress, lower self-esteem, and depression. It limits thinking and harms relationships with others.

- But we can learn to talk more positively to ourselves. We can reframe negative self-talk into encouraging self-talk. "I can't do this" could become "I can figure out how to do this." We can also choose more neutral language. "I hate this" might become "I'm annoyed by this."

- Also, new research shows that talking to ourselves in the third person is particularly effective. If instead of saying, "I'm so bad at this," I say, "Jaimie is so bad at this," it helps to distance me from the experience, and results are better. It seems weird at first, but with practice, it becomes a positive habit.

CARPE DIEM
The next time you catch yourself in negative self-talk,
flip it to something neutral or positive. Bonus points if you try
talking about yourself in the third person.

52.

TREAT YOURSELF WITH
SIMPLE PLEASURES

"The grass is greener where you water it."

— Neil Barringham

- What are the "little things" in life that make you feel happy, relaxed, grounded, grateful, or joyful in the moment? Pay attention to them, and incorporate them into every day. This is an important skill for everyone to develop, but especially those of us with a chronic illness.

- For me (Jaimie), these things include reading a book, enjoying a good movie, having coffee with a friend, writing or drawing in a journal, scrapbooking, spending time with pets, baking, singing, and dancing. For me (Alan), these things include spending time with my wife, hiking with my dogs, listening to music, watching the sunset, attending cars shows, and enjoying an interest in architecture and home design.

- Note that these "little things," when you add them all up, become the "big things." After all, life is essentially a series of moment-by-moment choices. When we choose to spend more of our moments on simple pleasures, our overall quality of life is enhanced.

- Also note that simple pleasures are often low-cost or even free, and require little effort. Our chronic illnesses do not prevent us from enjoying life.

CARPE DIEM
Intentionally incorporate at least one simple pleasure into this day.

53.

OBSERVE COMPLAINING

"Talking about our problems is our greatest addiction.
Break the habit. Talk about your joys."

— Rita Schiano

• Complaining about our chronic illnesses can be both good and bad. As we've been emphasizing, expressing our inner thoughts and feelings is good. Bottled-up, denied, and ignored feelings tend to fester into depression, anxiety, problems with intimacy, and other issues that make our lives worse, not better.

• But when does healthy expression become complaining? It's a question of audience, reciprocity, frequency, and intent.

• Some people are naturally good at listening without judgment to your thoughts and feelings. They are empathizers. Others will not be able to support you in this manner, but maybe they can in other ways, such as with practical help, entertainment, or socializing.

• Reciprocity means that if you are expressing painful thoughts and feelings to someone else, you should also be a good, active, nonjudgmental listener to them.

• Frequency is another consideration. Even skilled empathizers will fatigue if called on to empathize too often.

• Finally, and importantly, consider your intent. If your intent in expressing your feelings is to honor those feelings and give them momentum so they can soften and change, that is productive. If, however, your true intent is to find fault, criticize, or defend, your expressions may be counterproductive, both to yourself and to your relationship with the other person.

CARPE DIEM
Practice reciprocity in an important relationship today.

54.

FIND YOUR GRATITUDE

"Every day may not be good, but there is something good in every day."
— Unknown

- In the daily slog of chronic illness plus all our other commitments—work, family, homekeeping, pet care, financial, etc.—it can be hard to recognize the good in our lives.

- So we have to do it on purpose. Intentionally making time for gratitude each day is one of the best ways to give ourselves a dose of much-needed perspective and a dollop of happiness.

- Who and what are you grateful for in your life overall? Who and what are you grateful for in the past year? Who and what are you grateful for on this particular day? We can all learn to inventory our gratitude by making it an explicit task.

- To intentionally acknowledge their gratitude, some people meditate each morning on what they are grateful for. Others write a thank-you note or make a point of speaking a specific thank you aloud each day to someone in their lives. And some people make notes in a gratitude journal for a few minutes each night when they climb into bed.

CARPE DIEM
Spend the next five minutes expressing gratitude in some way.

55.

MAKE A PLAN FOR COPING WITH GRIEFBURSTS

"Life is not the way it is supposed to be. It is the way it is.
The way you cope with it is what makes the difference."

— Virginia Satir

• Sometimes our emotional response to our chronic illness in the heat of the moment—such as when we learn test results, experience a new or worsening symptom, or suddenly realize we can't participate in something important—overwhelms us.

• In such moments, strong feelings of loss, despair, sadness, and grief can knock us over like a powerful wave. We call this a "griefburst."

• During a griefburst, you might feel the need to cry, rage, or get yourself away from everyone else (or all three!).

• Griefbursts happen. You can't predict them, and you can't really control them either. All you can do is find ways to "be" with them in the now that work for you.

• Don't hesitate to try out different griefburst strategies. It might take some trial and error to find the crisis plans that work best for you.

CARPE DIEM

Now, in the calm of this moment, consider possible ways
you might "be" with your next griefburst.

56.

LEVERAGE THE LOVE LANGUAGES

"Being deeply loved by someone gives you strength,
while loving someone deeply gives you courage."

— Lao Tzu

- Chronic illness can make us feel overly dependent on others. We may feel needy, or we might feel guilty about monopolizing others' time. Or, conversely, we might avoid needing others in order to avoid these feelings!

- Regardless of where you fall on the dependence-on-others spectrum, we want you to know that it's healthy to connect with others in mutual empathy. In other words, relationships with other people are absolutely essential to a full, healthy life. And adult relationships are a two-way street: you help and care about me, and I'll help and care about you.

- Balance in relationships is key. You might need others to help you more with physical tasks than you are able to offer in return, for example, but if this is the case, you can balance the scales in other ways.

- The creator of the popular "love languages" concept, Dr. Gary Chapman, says there are five primary ways that humans feel cared for by others: receiving gifts, spending quality time together, hearing words of affirmation, being the beneficiary of acts of service, and experiencing physical touch. Each of us has a preferred love language. Working to understand and use the most effective love languages in your relationships with the people in your life will help balance and strengthen those relationships.

CARPE DIEM
Identify your primary love language, and ask someone close to you to identify theirs. This mutual understanding can help both of you.

57.

EMBRACE ENVY

"Health is a crown that the healthy wear, but only the sick can see it."
— Imam Shafi'ee

- Jealousy is when we feel threatened that someone we care about will be taken away from us by a competing person or circumstance. Envy, on the other hand, is when we feel that we lack something—possibly something we can see someone else has.

- Let's face it: chronic illness has a way of highlighting our lacks. What *don't* we have (or may not have in the future) because of our conditions? For some of us, the list is long.

- Like all feelings, envy is normal and natural. If we are feeling envious, it's because it's there to teach us something.

- So if and when you feel that prickle of envy, sit down with it. Invite it to speak to you. Ask it why it's there and what it really wants and needs. Empathize with it, and learn from it.

CARPE DIEM
What makes you feel envious? The next time you feel that pang
of envy, take it out for a walk or a cup of coffee.
Nurse it, and see what it has to teach you.

58.

IF YOU FEEL GUILT, FIND WAYS TO EXPRESS IT

"The guilt you feel finally comes to an end when you fully express how it came into your consciousness."
— Luke Garne

- As we've emphasized, all emotions are normal. If you're feeling something, it just means that you need to pay attention to it, work to name and understand it, and express it.

- In chronic illness, guilt, shame, and regret are common feelings. You may or may not experience feelings of guilt, but if you do, those feelings might arise because you aren't able to fulfill all of your perceived obligations, your care is costly (both in money and in time), or any number of other circumstances.

- The double-trouble with guilt often arises when we feel shame about our feelings of guilt, which simply creates weightier and weightier guilt.

- If you ever feel guilt, shame, or regret in connection with your chronic illness, please express those feelings out loud to others. Talk about your guilt. Allow yourself to be vulnerable and open in revealing your guilt. When you do, you will likely find understanding. Other people will often reveal guilt of their own. They will help you see that you are being too hard on yourself. And many will also forgive if forgiveness is needed.

- Exposing guilt to the light of day typically reveals it to be a much smaller monster than it seemed in the dark of our closets.

CARPE DIEM
If you harbor guilt, find some small way to expose
it to the light of day today.

59.

CHOOSE TO RISE ABOVE FEAR

*"Here is the world. Beautiful and terrible things will happen.
Don't be afraid."*

— Frederick Buechner

- Fear is a normal part of loss and uncertainty, but it's helpful to understand that fear is a biological response to perceived danger.

- In our bodies, perceived danger activates the evolutionary fight, flee, or freeze response, which has kept humankind alive for millennia. Our sympathetic nervous systems and adrenal-cortisol system set a cascade of physical responses in motion, activating nerve pathways and releasing stress hormones into the bloodstream.

- We have a natural tendency to fear both the unwanted and unknown outcomes of our illnesses. Our illnesses are perceived dangers, so our bodies activate the fear response.

- The true danger, however, is living in fear. Ongoing, stuck fear stresses our minds, bodies, hearts, and souls. While occasional bursts of fear are to be expected and met with self-compassion, constant fear actually harms us physically, cognitively, emotionally, socially, and spiritually.

- If you are often or always afraid, please ask your healthcare providers for help. Many therapies and techniques can ease fear. There is a combination out there that will work for you. You do not have to live in constant or pervasive fear. Only when your fear is under control will you be in a position to optimize meaning and joy.

CARPE DIEM
If you struggle with fear (or its close cousin, anxiety),
make an appointment with a counselor today.

60.

WORK THROUGH ANGER IN PRODUCTIVE WAYS

*"You will not be punished for your anger,
you will be punished by your anger."*
— Buddha

- Most of us with a chronic illness feel angry about it sometimes. It's frustrating, it's a pain (often literally), and it's damned unfair.

- Anger is a protest emotion. That means it's essentially a form of protesting something that is happening that we don't want to happen. Hate, blame, terror, resentment, rage, and jealousy are also protest emotions. And beneath them are usually helplessness, hurt, pain, and fear.

- There's nothing wrong with anger. It's normal and natural. But it is wrong to lash out when we're angry and hurt other people—or even hurt ourselves if we're physically acting out.

- We can instead learn to subdue and channel our anger in productive ways. The next few times you're angry, try a few different techniques. Go for a short walk. Turn on music and dance or sing. Close your eyes and breathe deeply. Meditate. Write in your journal. Wash the dishes. Vacuum the car. Often moving your body will not only help dissipate tense energy but also get something accomplished at the same time.

- And when you've calmed down a bit, don't forget to share your angry thoughts and feelings with someone who cares. Naming and discussing your anger will help you learn from it.

CARPE DIEM
If you're angry, try a new method of subduing and
channeling your anger today.

61.

ACKNOWLEDGE WHAT YOU CAN AND CANNOT CONTROL

*"Sometimes you will be in control of your illness,
and other times you'll sink into despair, and that's OK!
Freak out, forgive yourself, and try again tomorrow."*
— Kelly Hemingway

- So much of chronic illness is outside our control. We may be able to control our symptoms to some degree, through good self-care, but we can't make it go away, and we often can't stop flare-ups.

- In general, differentiating between what we can and cannot control is a helpful practice. We only have so much time and energy. It's better to spend them on things we can do something about.

- Here are some things we can control: our diets, our stress-management techniques, our participation in and compliance with healthcare, our daily schedules (to some extent, at least), the media and messages we take in, the amount of time we spend in front of screens, our outreach to friends and family, how we love others, our spiritual and creative tasks, our spending, our efforts at our jobs or other work, our focus on self-compassion, our gratitude.

- Here are some things we can't control: our bodies (not completely), what other people do and say (including our healthcare providers), world events.

- We only have so much time and energy. Let's spend them on things we can control.

CARPE DIEM
Make two lists: What I Can't Control and What I Can Control.

62.

MAKE A LIST OF THINGS YOU CAN'T DO

"Mostly it is loss which teaches us about the worth of things."
— Arthur Schopenhauer

- Things we can't do (but wish we could) as a result of our illnesses are among the losses we grieve. Stating them plainly helps us encounter and mourn them.

- As a result of my (Jaimie's) Type 1 diabetes, I can't leave the house without medical supplies and some source of sugar. I can't be careless about any substance that enters my body. I can't ignore the signs of low or high blood sugar. I can't be careless about my medical supplies and prescriptions. I can't be carefree.

- Whatever we feel about the items on this list is OK to feel. We might feel sad, mad, overwhelmed, guilty, or any number of things. And our feelings about them will probably change from week to week and year to year. What's more, the list will change as we get older and our life and illness circumstances change.

- When we acknowledge and allow ourselves to sit with our feelings of grief, we learn to integrate them into our lives. They are part of who we are. It may seem counterintuitive, but this befriending process actually helps lessen the pain over time.

- Now, move to the next Idea in this book and make a list of things you *can* do.

CARPE DIEM
Make that list, either in your head, on paper, or in a conversation with someone who cares. Allow yourself to grieve and mourn your "can'ts."

63.

NOW MAKE A LIST OF THINGS YOU *CAN* DO

---

*"Never let the things you cannot do prevent you
from doing the things you can."*
— Coach John Wooden

- Even though we may not be able to do everything we would like to do, there are still so many things we *can* do.

- Make a list of the things, big and little, that you appreciate being able to do. Include simple things, such as snuggling with your dog or singing along to your favorite songs, and more complex things, such as running a household, making holiday arrangements, or working on your hobbies. Also include things that you probably can and would like to do but have never tried. Write until you can't think of anything else. We bet your "can" list is longer than your "can't" list.

- Now circle the items on your "can" list that are most important to you.

- What did you circle? These are the things that give your life meaning. These are the things that spark hope and joy. These are the things that you should be intentionally incorporating more of into your everyday life.

CARPE DIEM
Pick one of the circled items and do it today.

64.

FLOAT ATOP UNCERTAINTY

*"The world is more magical, less predictable, more autonomous,
less controllable, more varied, less simple, more infinite,
less knowable, more wonderfully troubling than we could
have imagined being able to tolerate when we were young."*

— James Hollis

- Life is unpredictable. It's been said that uncertainty is the only certainty.

- For people with chronic illness, life can be especially unforeseeable. For one, many chronic illnesses fluctuate in severity and frequency of symptoms from month to month or even day to day. And for another, the future may be murky. Who knows what will be happening with our bodies and treatment options a few years from now?

- We can take good care of ourselves, but we can't completely control what happens to us. We can, however, work on controlling our responses to what happens to us.

- Picture yourself floating on a raft in the middle of the ocean. The raft is the support system you've built for yourself. It's your friends and family, your self-care practices, the assets you've built—financial, educational, spiritual, and more. When waves of change and challenge come along, the raft allows you to float.

- Yes, it can still get rocky up there on your raft, but you're still above water. Chaos may be reigning around you—even within your own body sometimes—but you're still floating.

CARPE DIEM

If uncertainty often makes you anxious or feel stressed,
take action today. Meditation and counseling are two good
tools for dealing with uncertainty.

65.

SOCIALIZE

"The 'I' in illness is isolation, and the crucial letters in wellness are 'we.'"
— Unknown

• People with naturally extroverted personalities tend to take care of this need without thought, but sometimes chronic illness shuts them down socially. If this is you, reach out to a close friend or family member and talk to them about your need to spend time with other people. Strategize ways to reconnect.

• People with naturally introverted personalities, on the other hand, are at risk for self-isolating, especially when chronic illness is part of the picture.

• Can you live without interacting with other people? Yes. Is it a good idea? No.

• Humans are social animals. Studies show that regular social contact keeps us physically and mentally healthier, lessens our risk of depression and anxiety, lengthens our lifespans, and makes us happier.

• Besides, face-to-face, close human relationships are what give our lives meaning, and that's what we're after in this book. Love is always the most important thing, and love requires social connections. So socialize away, even if it's with just a few special people.

CARPE DIEM
Make plans for some socializing today.

66.

LEARN TO NAME YOUR FEELINGS

"The emotion that can break your heart is sometimes the very one that heals it."

— Nicholas Sparks

- In the Introduction to this book, we talked about grief, which is the single name we give to all the many thoughts and feelings of loss we experience during our chronic-illness journey. It's normal and natural to feel frustrated and sad about having a chronic illness. It's OK to be angry.

- Learning to attune to, respect, and express our grief is an important part of our work. So is acknowledging each of the separate thoughts and feelings that comprise our grief.

- If I'm feeling out of sorts because I'm not physically able to do something I want to do today, for example, I might take a moment to sit with that feeling. What is it that I'm feeling, exactly? Am I angry? Disappointed? Jealous? Sad? Stinging over the injustice?

- When we're able to name our feeling(s), then we're better able to talk about them to others (or to ourselves, in our journals). We're more likely to experience self-awareness, which can lead to breakthrough self-understanding and productive change.

- Remember that feelings are not right or wrong. They simply are. We must allow ourselves to feel whatever it is we are feeling without judging ourselves. Befriending and getting to know our feelings normalizes them and helps soften them.

CARPE DIEM
What are you feeling right now, and why? Name it and befriend it.

67.

RECOGNIZE THE SIGNS OF CLINICAL DEPRESSION

- While it's normal to experience grief about the many losses that may result from your chronic illness, it's also important to learn to distinguish between the normal depression of grief and clinical depression.

- According to the National Institute of Mental Health, symptoms of clinical depression may include:

  - Difficulty concentrating, remembering details, and making decisions

  - Fatigue and decreased energy

  - Feelings of guilt, worthlessness, and/or helplessness

  - Feelings of hopelessness and/or pessimism

  - Insomnia, early-morning wakefulness, or excessive sleeping

  - Irritability, restlessness

  - Loss of interest in activities or hobbies once pleasurable, including sex

  - Overeating or appetite loss

  - Persistent aches or pains, headaches, cramps, or digestive problems that do not ease, even with treatment

  - Persistent sad, anxious, or "empty" feelings

  - Thoughts of suicide, suicide attempts

- Another way to think about the difference between grief and depression is to consider *how long the feelings last and to what extent your daily activities are impaired.* Grief softens over time and with active mourning; clinical depression does not. If you are clinically depressed, you may be unable to function day-to-day.

CARPE DIEM
If you are experiencing some of the symptoms listed above, make an appointment to see your primary-care physician or therapist today. It is not weakness but strength to acknowledge you need medical care. Drug and talk therapy may transform your life.

68.

GO AHEAD AND ASK WHY

"Life is an unanswered question, but let's still believe in the dignity and importance of the question."

— Tennessee Williams

- We talked about the universal need to search for meaning in Idea 10, but it's so important that we want to reiterate it here.

- Chronic illness is not fair. We didn't ask for it. We didn't deserve it. So why us?

- It's normal and natural to ask why. It's normal and natural to feel that we've been singled out or dealt a bad hand. It's normal and natural to question God or ask why bad things happen to good people. Speaking your why questions aloud to friends, family members, spiritual leaders, and others will help diminish their power over you.

- Along the way, though, it's also normal and natural to begin to feel movement in the asking process. Some people eventually develop beliefs about "why them"—beliefs that support them and make them feel a sense of purpose. Others begin to understand that there is no understanding—there is only standing under the mystery.

- So whenever you feel like asking why, by all means, ask. Answers can be overrated. The asking itself will help give you momentum to go forward.

CARPE DIEM
What are the most pressing "why" questions that you have?
Ask them aloud—to a friend, family member, coworker,
spiritual mentor, or healthcare provider—today.

69.

EMBRACE THE POWER
OF GOAL-SETTING

*"Greatness is not measured by what a man or woman accomplishes but by
the opposition he or she has overcome to reach his goals."*

— Dorothy Height

- Goal-setting is a close cousin to intention-setting (Idea 21).
  Both have the power to transform our lives.

- While intention-setting is about clarifying and rehearsing what we want
  to happen, goal-setting is more about establishing mile markers and
  measurable results. Intention-setting is more of a daily practice, while
  goal-setting is often longer-term.

- What are your goals this month or this year? Try writing down the
  three that you feel most passionate about.

- Once you've stated your goals, work backward and make a list of
  the incremental daily or weekly steps that you would need to take to
  achieve at least one of the goals. Add them to your calendar or to-do
  list.

- Make yourself accountable to your goals by working with a
  responsibility partner—a friend or family member who is also
  committed to working on a goal of their own. You can provide each
  other encouragement and support along the way.

CARPE DIEM
Plan out a goal today, and share it with someone else.

70.

CLAIM YOUR HUMANITY

"Do I contradict myself? Very well then, I contradict myself.
I am large. I contain multitudes."

— Walt Whitman

- Each of us is a unique human being challenged by unique challenges, blessed by unique blessings, and living in unique and ever-changing circumstances. This is true of every single person—those who have a chronic illness and those who do not.

- To be a human being is to be a drop in the ocean of humanity.

- To claim our humanity means to acknowledge and embrace the reality that our lives are ephemeral and we do not have complete control over them. We're here for a short, wild ride, then we're gone.

- To claim our humanity also means to acknowledge that our chronic illnesses are not who we are but instead part of who we are. Each of us is so many different, changing, and sometimes contradictory things. Each of us is a multitude unto ourself.

- We're so small and insignificant in the scheme of human history, yet we're miraculous, singular individuals different from anyone who has ever lived before. To claim our humanity means to embrace this paradox.

CARPE DIEM
Stargaze tonight, and while you're marveling at the stars, think about your place in humanity and in the universe.

71.

CULTIVATE PATIENCE

"Patience and perseverance have a magical effect before which difficulties disappear and obstacles vanish."

— John Quincy Adams

- Patience is the art of sitting in the moment with what is and practicing non-attachment to outcome.

- When we're impatient, we're restlessly waiting for something we want to happen, right? We're allowing a hoped-for future to negatively affect our now.

- Patience is an especially important habit to cultivate in chronic illness because time schedules are often waylaid by symptoms and care protocols. Life often becomes necessarily slower with chronic illness. We can choose to embrace this as a good thing.

- As we said, patience is a habit. It is a practice. It is not a hardwired personality trait. Yes, you've developed patience or impatience habits over the course of your life so far, but those habits can be changed.

- Any practices that help you live in the now will help you cultivate patience, such as meditation, bracketing concerns for a prearranged time, enjoying nature, and engaged presence with someone loved.

CARPE DIEM

Today, if you notice yourself getting impatient, make an intentional choice to experience and accept the moment as it is.

72.

SIMPLIFY

"Simplicity is nature's first step, and the last of art."

— Philip James Bailey

- Throughout human history, people have had to cope with scarcity—not enough food, not enough resources, not enough recreation. Today, though, while there are still certainly pockets of scarcity, more and more people are having to cope with overabundance instead. Too much food, too many resources, too many recreational choices.

- Simplifying our lives helps us get back to that just-right balance between not enough and too much. When we clear excess things and activities from our homes and our lives, we can often find the peace and joy of mindful living.

- You may have heard of FOMO, which is short for the Fear Of Missing Out. FOMO is that modern-day feeling that you're missing out on internet memes, political news, good TV shows, what your friends are doing, and more if you're not constantly searching, reading, doing, and trying to keep up. But an even newer trend is JOMO, or the Joy Of Missing Out. JOMO celebrates living in the now without concern for what everyone else is reading, watching, or doing.

- There's joy to be found in simplicity and embracing the fullness of each moment, no matter what that moment contains (or doesn't contain). There's fulfillment to be found in the just-right balance between not enough and too much.

CARPE DIEM

Simplify your free time today by stepping away from your computer, tablet, TV, and phone, and enjoying a non-digital pleasure.

73.

EXPLORE WHAT YOU CAN EXPLORE

"So, do it. Decide. Is this the life you want to live?
Is this the person you want to love? Is this the best you can be?
Can you be stronger? Kinder? More compassionate?
Decide. Breathe in. Breathe out and decide."

— Grey's Anatomy

- Each of us comes to this book on chronic illness with unique life experiences, circumstances, personalities, strengths, and challenges. Despite our differences, we have many things in common.

- One thing we have in common is the need to continually consider and push our own boundaries. Why?

- Whenever we opt to stay only within our comfort zones, we're at risk for dying while we're alive. It's too easy to place false limits on our abilities, our knowledge, and our hopes and dreams. When we tell ourselves, "I do this, but I don't do that," we're lopping off potential joys and meaning.

- We're not saying that anyone can do anything. That's just not true. We're also not saying that we constantly have to be trying new things to live our best lives. That's silly.

- What we *are* saying is that if our divine sparks glow a little more brightly when we consider a certain person, place, or activity—or if we harbor "I've always wanted to…," bucket-list desires—that means we're meant to explore them. Many of us need to push our own boundaries and take scary steps to venture into those explorations. Here we go.

CARPE DIEM
Fill in the blank: I've always wanted to _____.
Whatever it is, explore it today.

74.

MAKE A TO-DO LIST FOR DAYS YOU'RE DISCOURAGED

"Planning is bringing the future into the present so that you can do something about it now."
— Alan Lakein

- When we're sick of being sick, it's understandable to feel discouraged. Down days are part of the human experience for everyone, but chronic illness can tip the scales too often and too much.

- You know how groups make plans and do practice drills in anticipation of crises? We can and should do the same thing—in advance—for the discouraging days we know will come. So sit down on a good day and make a plan for your next bad day. Give yourself a few options in each of the following categories: wallow, soothe, connect, and foster hope.

- Wallowing means allowing yourself to acknowledge, feel, and express your discouragement. Wallowing is good because it's honest. Potential wallowing activities for your to-do list include crying, ruminating, journaling, and complaining to understanding others.

- Soothing activities are those that comfort us. What comforts you? Possible activities for this section of your crisis list include taking a bath, eating comfort food, watching your favorite movie, or cuddling with your pet.

- Connecting with others also combats despair. Note things like calling a friend, sharing a meal with a loved one, or reaching out via social media in this section of your plan.

- Finally, jot down at least several activities that make you hopeful about the future. These might include making fun plans for tomorrow or next week, or setting an achievable short-term goal.

CARPE DIEM
On your next down day, pull out this to-do list. Choose at least one activity from each of the four categories and give them a try. Notice how you feel when you've completed them.

75.

REACH OUT

"The most important thing I think we need to remember is that we're a work in progress. Do not be ashamed or afraid to ask for help."

— Carnie Wilson

- Chronic illness is often an isolating experience, but human beings are social creatures. It is our connections with others that give our life the fullest of meaning.

- Raise your hand if you've ever thought, "I don't want to burden other people with my problems." No doubt there are a lot of hands in the air. But here's the thing: everyone has problems. The people you don't want to burden almost certainly need a listening ear and a supportive shoulder too.

- Don't be afraid to ask for help. You may need actual physical help, maybe with transportation or everyday chores. Or perhaps you could use a hand with paperwork or financial matters. And most of all, you really do need others who will listen without judgment and offer empathy and kindness.

- Don't forget to offer help in return. After all, relationships are two-way streets, and they are usually strongest when they are balanced and equal. Learn to be a good listener and supporter. And be a pitcher-inner in whatever ways you can.

- We're fortunate that modern technology allows us to reach out in a variety of ways. Keeping in touch with others via texts, phone calls, Skype, social media, and online forums doesn't replace the need for face-to-face human contact, but it can be a good supplement. Social media also allows those of us with chronic illness to find and communicate with others with the same condition, who are going through similar struggles and frustrations.

CARPE DIEM
Right now, reach out to someone you haven't connected with in a while but have been meaning to. Send a text, make a call, or pop in. Notice how it makes you feel.

76.

GO TO "THIN PLACES"

"Spiritual and metaphysical health is inextricably linked to physical health."
— Dr. Morris Hyman

- In the Celtic tradition, "thin places" are spots where the separation between the physical world and the spiritual world seems tenuous.

- They are places where the veil between heaven and earth, between the holy and the everyday, are so thin that when we are near them, we intuitively sense the timeless, boundless spiritual world.

- Thin places are usually outdoors, often where water and land meet or land and sky come together. We might find thin places on a riverbank, a beach, or a mountaintop.

- Sacred spots—such as cathedrals, mosques, temples, memorials, cemeteries—are also often thin places. But really, wherever you feel a sense of otherworldly transcendence is a thin place for you, though it may not be for someone else.

- Thin places are good destinations for considering the big questions of life and attuning to our divine sparks. They're also good places to mourn our losses, and find hope and healing.

CARPE DIEM
Spend time in a thin place today.

77.

FIND A SPIRITUAL HOME

*"Just as a candle cannot burn without fire, men cannot
live without a spiritual life."*
— Buddha

- Giving daily time and attention to our spirituality is just as important as caring for our bodies. Why? Because that's where purpose and meaning live.

- As we've said, different people nurture their spirits in different ways. Some participate in religious activities. Some meditate, garden, make art, or spend time in nature.

- No matter how you feed your spirit, you may find it helpful to establish a spiritual home. This is a particular, physical place where you can go whenever you need to feel spiritually grounded. It might be a church, synagogue, mosque, temple, park, beach, forest, meadow, riverbank, or mountain peak. Going there is essentially a shortcut to feeling a connection with the divine.

- Consider choosing a place near your home, so you can go there often. You can even create a spiritual home within your house, by setting up a room or an area specially for spiritual contemplation.

CARPE DIEM
Today, visit or begin your quest to find your spiritual home.

78.

SANDWICH MEANING INTO EACH DAY

"Health is a large word. It embraces not the body only but the mind and spirit as well. Not today's pain or pleasure alone, but the whole being and outlook."

— James H. West

- What are some things that give your life meaning? What brings you a sense of purpose, satisfaction, accomplishment, connection, or joy? What are the "small things" in your days and weeks that make you feel contented, loved, or happy?

- Whatever those things are for you, you can intentionally schedule them into each day.

- Think of your day like a sandwich. You get to choose how to layer it. To make your sandwich hold together and sustain you, you might need to include a few ingredients you don't love—maybe housecleaning or some aspects of your job, for example. But you also get to tuck in bits of your favorites, creating, overall, a delectable sandwich.

- If you're a bacon person, you might think of meaning as the bacon in your daily sandwich. (If you're not a bacon person, that's OK. Just pick *your* favorite sandwich topping for this metaphor!) No matter what else is going on with that sandwich, the bacon makes it pretty delicious, right? The same thing happens when you layer meaningful activities and moments into your day. No matter what else is going on in your life, those special bits—even just a sprinkling—can make it delicious.

CARPE DIEM
With intention, sandwich some meaning into this day.

79.

SHARE YOUR GIFTS

"Don't ask what the world needs. Ask what makes you come alive, and go do it. Because what the world needs is people who have come alive."
— Howard Thurman

- Whether you realize it or not, you have gifts. Everyone does. We all have things we're naturally good at.

- Often our gifts seem like givens to us. They're no big deal. The effortlessness with which we accomplish them can make us overlook or undervalue them.

- What have people told you you're good at? What have others come to you for help with over the years? In a group setting, what are you typically asked or relied upon to contribute? These things are your gifts.

- Those of us with chronic illness have losses, yes, but we also have gains. When we share those positives with others, we are interacting with the world in meaningful ways. We are contributing. We are making a difference.

- Identify your gifts then share them. That simple statement is a significant part of what it means to live your best life.

CARPE DIEM
Today, identify a gift and share it.

80.

HAVE A CHOICE?
CHOOSE MEANING

*"I often say now I don't have any choice whether
I have Parkinson's, but surrounding that non-choice is
a million other choices that I can make."*

— Michael J. Fox

- Every day, every hour, every moment, we have choices. What should I do next? What should I do *right now*?

- With or without chronic illness, living our best lives means making good choices, day to day, hour to hour, moment to moment.

- While a million factors may weigh on any given choice we have to make in the moment, we'd like to advocate for one factor weighing more heavily than all the others, and that's *meaning*.

- Let's say you have a relatively free afternoon. There are many things you may need to do to continue living a healthy, stable life, such as shopping for nutritious food, exercising, paying bills, etc. OK. All of those requirements are meaningful because without them you can't possibly live well. Once your baseline needs are taken care of, though, what should you do with the rest of the free time? We hope you'll choose higher-level meaning.

- Choosing meaning means purposefully allocating time for the people and activities most important to you. For example, watching TV may or may not be choosing meaning for you, but watching TV with a close friend probably is. Spending money on a luxury vehicle may or may not be choosing meaning for you, but saving money to travel somewhere you've always wanted to go probably is.

CARPE DIEM
When you have a choice to make today, choose meaning.

81.

INDULGE YOUR CREATURE COMFORTS

"There is a comfort in rituals, and rituals provide a framework for stability when you are trying to find answers."
— Deborah Norville

- Our bodies like to be comfortable and cozy. Providing them with what they need to feel this way as much as possible is a big part of our job as self-caregivers. When our bodies are comfy and cozy, we're more likely to have the energy and attention spans to act on our cognitive, emotional, social, and spiritual needs.

- Conversely, it's much harder to connect with our higher-level needs when we're experiencing physical discomfort. When we indulge our physical needs first, the rest is able to follow.

- Have you heard of the Danish concept of *hygge*? Pronounced HEW-guh, the term means, according to the *Oxford Dictionary*, "a quality of coziness and comfortable conviviality that engenders a feeling of contentment or wellbeing."

- Whatever creates that sense of hygge for you, add it to your daily routines. Comfy shoes, a cozy shirt or jacket, your favorite mug, candles, a tidy room, a leather chair, a special candy or food—layer in a number of elements that make you feel comfortable, relaxed, and well cared-for.

CARPE DIEM
Hygge your day today.

82.

ASK YOURSELF, "WHAT SHOULD I DO?"

"Intuition is seeing with the soul."

— Dean Koontz

- As we actively work to live our best lives with chronic illness, we're learning to pay close and careful attention to our bodies, our minds, our hearts, and our spirits.

- In other words, we're learning to listen to ourselves. We're learning to honor and attend to our needs and desires, no matter how quiet and subtle they may be.

- We can bring this enhanced capacity to tune into our internal wisdom to all our encounters and decisions. Whenever we're at a crossroads, big or small, we can ask ourselves, "What should I do?"

- Our internal wisdom is also called our intuition or "gut instinct." When we ask ourselves, "What should I do?", we're making a gut check. We're using our intuition to help us decide our best path.

- When we learn to trust and rely on our intuition, our lives become simpler and more carefree. We don't have to agonize; we just have to ask and follow.

CARPE DIEM
Today, ask your intuition, "What should I do?"

83.

SPEND TIME WITH AT LEAST ONE "WOW" EVERY DAY

"Life is either a daring adventure or nothing at all."
— Helen Keller

- Sometimes life feels "blah." We may be stuck in a rut or struggling to just manage our chronic illnesses every day. Maybe work or daily routines seem lifeless. Maybe the weather is dreary, and maybe our souls are drearier.

- In this age of information overload, we have ample opportunity to discover tidbits online or in the media that amaze and delight us. There are so many fantastic things in this world! Trouble is, the firehose of delight that is the internet comes at us in such a deluge that we often end up feeling numb and over-stimulated instead of awed.

- The same thing can happen with our real, in-person lives. Amazing people, things, and occurrences constantly surround us, but we're often blind to them because of their familiarity.

- How about we intentionally look for and reflect on one single "wow" each day? Instead of rushing past all the amazing things and people we see and encounter, what if we stop and spend time with one of them? For example, what if we had an intimate, meaningful, non-distracted, face-to-face discussion with one person we care about? What if we stopped to not only smell one rose but give it our undivided attention and curiosity for a while?

- The habit of selecting and giving one single "wow" our full attention for perhaps 30 minutes a day has the power to change our whole life experience.

CARPE DIEM

Pick a "wow" and give it your full attention for half an hour today.

84.

TAKE BABY STEPS

"Sometimes the smallest step in the right direction ends up being the biggest step of your life. Tiptoe if you must, but take a step."

— Naeem Callaway

- We often hear that life isn't about the goals or results we achieve—it's about the journey.

- But here's the thing: We're not really on a journey unless we're moving. Right?

- We've talked about setting intentions and goals, and we do believe those practices are essential to moving in the directions your soul is whispering you to take. Yet the most essential thing of all is to keep moving.

- When we feel stuck, it's often because we're doing the same unsatisfying things over and over again. That's not really moving. That's stasis. That's spinning in a circle.

- But every day that we take baby steps in the direction of intention, desire, joy, purpose, or meaning, we're moving. Who knows where we'll end up, but we're moving. And *that* is what the journey is all about.

CARPE DIEM
Feeling stuck? Take one step in the direction of intention, desire, joy, purpose, or meaning today.

85.

BE A JOY DETECTIVE

"Be soft. Do not let the world make you hard. Do not let the pain make you hate. Do not let the bitterness steal sweetness. Take pride that even though the rest of the world may disagree, you still believe it to be a beautiful place."

— Iain S. Thomas

- When joy isn't easy to find, don your detective hat.

- What does it mean to be a detective? If means to actively, determinedly, and carefully go looking for something.

- Detectives can't always predict where they'll discover a break in the case, but they have some tried and true places to look. You, too, have some tried and true places, people, or activities where you often find joy. Go to your old reliables.

- If you're not finding joy in your old reliables, you'll need to keep looking. Follow up on possible clues and suspicions about new ways of discovering joy. Interview other people about how they find joy. Read joyful books, watch joyful movies, listen to joyful stories.

- Remember that joy isn't a single path leading to one destination. It's a daily, mindful habit composed of infinite paths and places. It can be found anywhere at any time, as long as you're willing to actively, determinedly, and carefully look for it.

CARPE DIEM
Go looking for joy today.

86.

RESPOND TO COMMENTS WITH HONESTY AND GRACE

"Maybe life isn't about avoiding the bruises.
Maybe it's about collecting the scars to prove that we showed up for it."
— Hannah Brencher

- Sometimes others may say ignorant, hurtful things to those of us with chronic illness. They might essentially blame us for our own diseases. They may imply we're lazy or fakers or poor caretakers of our own bodies. They might ask overly invasive questions or assume we're helpless or dumb.

- First, we can be honest. It is almost always the best policy. When someone says something inaccurate about us, we can correct them. Ideally our correction will be calm and factual. Education and patience can help change the minds and hearts of others.

- Second, we can acknowledge our feelings. When we are hurt, we can and should say so. We can practice naming our feelings, ideally without reciprocal blaming and tit-for-tat hurtfulness. We might say, "I feel hurt to be thought of as lazy. My energy is just naturally limited by my illness."

- And third, we can try to remember that what other people say is really about them, not about us. They are typically offering judgments based on their own fears and issues. It's hard to have grace when others say ignorant, hurtful things, but it's worth continuing to try. Grace makes our lives—and our world—better.

CARPE DIEM

The next time someone makes a hurtful comment or judgment about your chronic illness, stop for a moment and consider responding differently than you might have before.

87.

BE THE TORTOISE

*"If you can't fly then run, if you can't run then walk,
if you can't walk then crawl, but whatever you do,
you have to keep moving forward."*

— Martin Luther King, Jr.

- You remember Aesop's fable of the tortoise and the hare. The tortoise, who'd grown tired of the hare's bragging, challenged the hare to a race. The faster hare immediately sped ahead but then, overconfident, stopped midway to take a nap. The slow-but-steady tortoise crossed the finish line first.

- Many of us with chronic illness can relate to the tortoise. We may not have the energy or the speed to race ahead. We may be slow and plodding. And despite our slow pace, we may still have to take rests along the way.

- But nevertheless, slow and steady can get us where we want to go. If we use our potentially limited energy to inch ourselves forward little by little, bit by bit, day by day, we can still achieve meaningful goals.

- Whatever your natural, necessary pace these days, it's counterproductive to fight it or get overly discouraged by it. Instead, work with your pace and accommodate its unique needs, strengths, and limitations. As long as you keep going, it will get you across the finish line.

CARPE DIEM
Embrace your natural, necessary pace today.

88.

EMBRACE WABI-SABI

"Pared down to its barest essence, wabi-sabi is the Japanese art of finding beauty in imperfection and profundity in nature, of accepting the natural cycle of growth, decay, and death. It is simple, slow, and uncluttered—and it reveres authenticity above all."

— Tadao Ando

- Those of us with chronic illness are broken. We're imperfect. We have definite physical and sometimes cognitive and emotional flaws.

- But wait a second! Before you get angry about these provocative claims, consider that: a) *everyone* is imperfect and flawed, and b) our imperfections are what make each of us who we are.

- The Japanese Zen Buddhist philosophy called *wabi-sabi* cherishes the wisdom and beauty of imperfection and brokenness. Our favorite chipped mug, a worn sweater our grandmother knitted for us, the lines on our aging faces— all of these are wabi-sabi.

- In honor of this belief, some craftsmen practice an ancient art called *kintsugi,* which means "golden joinery." Kintsugi artists take broken pottery and china and join the fragments together with an epoxy that contains gold. The technique draws attention to and celebrates the imperfections.

- Yes, we are wabi-sabi, and so is everyone else. Whenever we see, feel, or experience brokenness or imperfection, in ourselves or in someone else, we are reminded to marvel at the variety and the authenticity—which is almost always, as it turns out, more interesting and perfect than perfect is.

CARPE DIEM
When you notice brokenness or imperfection today,
in yourself or someone else, choose to celebrate the flaw rather
than give in to anger, disappointment, or fear.

89.

REVEL IN THE BLESSINGS
OF THIS MOMENT

*"Thank you, dear God, for this good life, and forgive us
if we do not love it enough."*

— Garrison Keillor

- Have you ever noticed that even when things are going well, our minds tend to occupy themselves with more wanting?

- Say you're in a movie theater, waiting for a film you've been excited about to start. You've got good seats. You've got popcorn and your favorite beverage. You're sitting next to someone you enjoy going to movies with. Then you remember that chocolate bar in your cupboard at home. You should have brought it with you! Dang. A pang of disappointment pricks the moment.

- This no-win trap of *always wanting* may be human nature, but it's also something we can work to overcome.

- When we catch ourselves wanting, we can intentionally turn our attention to what we already have in that moment. We can silently and mindfully inventory our blessings then and there. We can even express our gratitude about those blessings by telling someone else about them, praying thanks about them, or making notes in a gratitude journal.

- Learning to revel in and be grateful for the blessings of the moment helps us live mindfully and more joyfully, especially on days when things aren't going as well as we'd hoped.

CARPE DIEM
Today, when you catch yourself wanting, mindfully turn your
attention to the blessings of the moment instead.

90.

MAKE A NOT-TO-DO LIST

"You don't have to do much to belong to yourself. All you have to do is get rid of all the things that don't make you feel true to yourself."

— Dr. Prem Jagyasi

- We all have a lot to do, and to-do lists help us remember important tasks. They're a useful little tool, because often, when we neglect to do something essential in a timely fashion, like pay the electricity bill, the consequences are often much more time-consuming and annoying to deal with than if we'd just taken care of the task in the first place.

- But have you ever made a not-to-do list? Turns out it's another little tool that can be a game-changer.

- Think about all the non-essential tasks and commitments you have on your plate. Are there any you don't enjoy or have the energy for anymore? If so, those might belong on your not-to-do list. It's self-compassionate to drop activities that no longer serve you well.

- What about physical, cognitive, emotional, social, or spiritual habits that harm, discourage, or numb you in some way? Those go on the not-do-list too.

CARPE DIEM
Make yourself a to-do list for today, then make a not-to-do list.
Follow both.

91.

WHEN YOU WANT TO
GIVE UP, DON'T

*"If opening your eyes, or getting out of bed, or holding a spoon,
or combing your hair is the daunting Mount Everest
you climb today, that is OK."*

— Carmen Ambrosio

- Discouragement and even despair are understandable in chronic illness. Human life is often hard, but life with chronic illness can sometimes seem intolerable.

- If you ever want to give up, look for inspiration. Talk to people who make you feel better. Find true stories that give you hope. Turn to activities that make you laugh.

- Remember the lead character in the animated Pixar movie *Finding Dory*? When the going got tough, she repeated this mantra to herself: Just keep swimming.

- Always remember that life happens one day at a time. Tomorrow will not be exactly the same as today, especially if you are reaching out to others and proactively finding ways to engage that give you hope and purpose.

- And some days or even weeks may simply be Mulligans. When you need to crawl back into bed and do nothing but grieve and survive, that's OK too. On those days, knowing that your time-out is temporary is enough.

CARPE DIEM
Make a list of ideas: Things I should do when I want to give up.

92.

ROLL WITH THE PUNCHES

"You have been told that, even like a chain,
you are as weak as your weakest link. This is but half the truth.
You are also as strong as your strongest link."
— Kahlil Gibran

- Chronic illness is often unpredictable. We may not know in advance how we'll feel tomorrow or what may happen next week.

- It's natural to feel frustrated or stymied by this uncertainty. But it's also possible to cultivate our own flexibility and resilience.

- We can't always control what happens, but we can control our responses to what happens. When we're frustrated, we can acknowledge our frustration then turn our attention to our best alternative course of action.

- When we think, "Ugh, I'm so mad/disappointed," we can intentionally follow that thought with, "OK, what's my best path today?" Sometimes really nice, unexpected opportunities present themselves when we choose to make this two-step thought pattern a habit.

- The idea isn't to deny our anger or frustration but rather to give them the attention they're asking for, and then, even as we're embracing those normal feelings, nurture our flexibility and resilience. It's not either/or. It's both.

CARPE DIEM
The next time you feel that twinge of frustration or disappointment,
acknowledge it, express it, and then ask yourself,
"OK, what's my best path now?"

93.

BE A KID AGAIN

*"To be more childlike, you don't have to give up being an adult.
The fully integrated person is capable of being both an adult
and a child simultaneously. Recapture the feelings of wide-eyed
excitement, spontaneous appreciation, cutting loose, and being full
of awe and wonder at this magnificent universe."*

— Wayne Dyer

- When life with chronic illness weighs us down, allowing the kid inside of us to take charge for a while can lift us up.

- What does it mean to "be a kid"? It means playing. It means being silly. It means not worrying. It means finding the good and the joy in every moment.

- What gives you an inexplicable burst of joy every time you see it or do it? What did you love as a child but haven't experienced lately? What's just plain fun to you? What are your favorite indulgences —preferably the most childlike ones?

- Chronic illness is often so serious. Finding ways to be a kid again regularly can lighten our lives, providing balance and some much-needed fun.

CARPE DIEM
Do something decidedly childlike today.

94.

IDENTIFY YOUR CHAMPIONS

"Choose people who lift you up."

— Michelle Obama

- In Idea 20 we talked about the rule of thirds: roughly a third of the people in your life will be helpful to you, a third will be neutral, and a third will be harmful. When you're struggling with your chronic illness, it's important to identify and spend time with the first third.

- Among the first third are special individuals who are your champions. They are the people who believe in you no matter what and would even lay down their lives for you if necessary.

- Your champions are your biggest cheerleaders and your most ardent fans. They're not necessarily perfect human beings—but they're perfectly supportive of you. Most of us have one champion. Those of us who are lucky might have two or three throughout the course of our lives.

- Who is your champion? Identify them now. Being clear in your own mind about who your champions are will help you remember whom to turn to when you need immediate, no-questions-asked support.

CARPE DIEM
Write a thank-you note to your champion(s) today.
Express the depths of your gratitude for the role they have played in your life so far as well as your hopes for a continued meaningful relationship in the months and years to come.

95.

STAND UNDER THE MYSTERY

"The mystery of life isn't a problem to solve but a reality to experience."
— Frank Herbert

- Whenever we experience suffering in life, it's normal to wonder and ask "why." In fact, "searching for meaning" is so universal that it is one of the six needs of mourning (need 5, Idea 10).

- When we are affected by a chronic illness, it's natural for us to want to understand. Our brains and our hearts often clamor for answers. Why us? Why this condition? Why now? Why, why, why?

- If such questions are welling up within us, that means we need to ask them. Expressing our thoughts and feelings is always the right path.

- But just because we ask such questions doesn't mean we'll find answers. It's the asking that's important.

- Instead of finding understanding, we might be on a path to learning to "stand under" the mystery. After all, for many of us the biggest "whys" of human existence don't have certain answers. They only have questioning and pondering. Standing under the mystery is a worthy goal in and of itself.

CARPE DIEM
Take time to ponder mystery (of your life, of your feelings for someone else, of the universe, or anything you want) today.

96.

WRITE A LETTER TO YOUR BODY

"She resented her body's betrayal. She still couldn't express how insecure it made her, how she lived on a precipice. The most basic parts of her could fail, and there was nothing she could do to stop it."

— Zoje Stage

- Our bodies *are* us, and yet they're separate from us. We live inside them, and we try to take care of them, but they often behave in ways we cannot control and do not like. It can be a frustrating paradox.

- How do you feel about your body right now? Expressing those feelings is good for your soul. So why not share them in the form of a letter?

- Writing a letter to your body is a process that invites you to clarify your thoughts and feelings. Working toward this clarity will help you become a better body-listener and strengthen your relationship with your body, as odd as that sounds.

- Tell your body why you're frustrated or angry with it. But also tell your body about all the ways you appreciate and are grateful for it.

- Becoming your body's empathetic friend and loyal advocate is the goal. After all, you're in this together.

CARPE DIEM
Write the letter today.

97.

SHAKE THINGS UP

"Most of the important things in the world have been accomplished by people who have kept on trying when there seemed to be no hope at all."

— Dale Carnegie

- The "chronic" in "chronic illness" is a significant part of our challenge. It's not short term. In fact, it may well be forever.

- Because our illnesses are something we have to live with and deal with every single day, we can be more susceptible to getting into ruts in our daily lives. Complacency can set in. We may find ourselves growing bored, irritable, or hopeless if our days are too uniform or tedious.

- When we're feeling these things, that's when it's time to shake things up. We do have significant control over our daily lives. Let's exert it.

- Here are just a few of the things we can "shake up" at any time: our clothing, our meals, what we view on TV, the websites we visit, the route we take to work or the doctor's office, the people we spend time with, our spiritual practices, our sleep habits, and so many more.

- Change is invigorating. It has the power to wake us up to life.

CARPE DIEM
Shake something in your life out of complacency today.

98.

SEARCH FOR A NEW NORMAL

"Courage doesn't always roar. Sometimes courage is the quiet voice at the end of the day saying, 'I will try again tomorrow.'"

— Mary Anne Radmacher

- The "Before" we talked about in Idea 12 is gone, and we mourn its passage. Now we're living in After, and we're challenged to create a "new normal."

- With chronic illness, we are often "stuck" with certain aspects of our physical conditions or limitations as well as our daily care. There are certain things we might not be able to do, and there are certain things we might have to do, such as take medication or get a certain amount of rest.

- So, our new normal includes these realities. But they're not the entirety of our new normal.

- We have the power to continue to search for and create a new normal in which we routinely experience a sense of meaning and purpose. Our new normal can and should also include love, hope, and joy.

- We may have been dealt a bad hand, but we're not out of the game. No siree. In our ongoing search for our best lives, we are finding ways to make our new normal as meaningful as possible.

CARPE DIEM
Do one small thing today to search for and create a new normal that builds in meaning and purpose.

99.

START TODAY

"Life is not easy, especially when you plan on achieving something worthwhile. Don't take the easy way out. Do something extraordinary."
— Maria Robinson

- When it comes to taking steps toward living our best lives, there's no time like the present.

- Studies show that it takes 21 days to establish a new habit and 90 days to turn that habit into a lifestyle. So when we start something today, in just three weeks it will likely be a habit, and in three months it will be an intrinsic part of who we are.

- There are so many things we can start today! If we're not exercising already, we may be able to take a five-minute walk or complete a five-minute chair-yoga session. We can check out a library book on a topic we're interested in. We can start a gratitude journal. We can try cooking a new healthy recipe. We can call a friend we've been meaning to reconnect with. We can schedule an appointment with a counselor or new healthcare provider. We can wash our sheets and make our bed. We can try meditating. We can make simple plans with a special loved one. Pick one or several!

- What small step could you take today that would make you feel like you've accomplished something? Do that. Then tomorrow, do another one.

CARPE DIEM
Start one small thing in one small way today.

100.

MAKE A MILLION

"If a little dreaming is dangerous, the cure for it is not to dream less but to dream more, to dream all the time."

— Marcel Proust

- What do you wish you had in abundance in your life? Get started on making a million.

- Sure, a million dollars might be nice, but do you know what would be nicer? A million smiles. A million embraces. A million hopes. A million joyful moments. A million dreams.

- Training ourselves to notice, count, and foster more of these little miracles as they happen is where we find meaning and live our best lives.

- A single year contains more than 31 million seconds, or half a million minutes. We can get a good jump on making a million in the year to come. We know *we're* eager to get started. How about you?

CARPE DIEM
Whatever you deep-down, truly desire to make a million of,
get started today.

A FINAL WORD

Chronic illness is a challenge none of us would choose for ourselves or our loved ones. It's not something we can deny, ignore, or wish away. It doesn't care if we can't do what we want to do or if we have to miss important life events. It's indifferent to the losses it causes in our lives. It can be unkind, and it often hurts.

But at the same time, chronic illness has been a gift. It's taught us what's truly important. It's made us more resilient and more self-compassionate. It's revealed to us the wonder of living in the now. And even as it's forcing us to adjust our expectations and deal with more loss, it's showing us that we can lay claim to a life of meaning, purpose, and joy nonetheless.

We hope the ideas in this book help you embrace and mourn your chronic-illness grief.

We hope you are surrounded by the love and care of others, and we hope you let them in whenever they knock.

We hope you look for beauty even in the ugliest moments.

We hope you find hope when you need it.

We hope you nurture your spirit in ways that bring you closer to your self and to God.

We hope you live with purpose and love each and every day of your life.

We hope you embrace what your life journey has been teaching you.

We hope you find untapped stores of compassion and strength inside yourself so that you can be kind to yourself as well as help others in need.

We hope you come to a place where you are ready to unwrap the gifts of chronic illness.

Blessings to you as you continue to explore your lessons learned, questions asked, and choices made.

We wish you peace and joy.

THE CHRONIC-ILLNESS
BILL OF RIGHTS

Ten Self-Compassionate Principles

Though you should reach out to others throughout your chronic-illness journey, you should not feel obligated to accept the unhelpful responses you may receive from some people. You are the expert of your experience, and you have certain rights no one can take away from you.

1. **You have the right to your own story about chronic illness.** You have your own unique experience with your chronic illness. You have the right to tell your story and express your feelings in your own unique way.

2. **You have the right to grieve and mourn your chronic illness as a significant loss.** Chronic illness creates many losses from the moment of diagnosis. Depending on what kind of chronic illness you have, these may include loss of mobility, loss of feeling, loss of energy, loss of independence, loss of confidence, loss of hope, and many more. It is your right to grieve and mourn every loss that comes with your chronic-illness grief.

3. **You have the right to feel a range of emotions regarding your illness.**
   You may feel shock, dismay, despair, anger, frustration, sadness, fear and many other emotions. Chronic illness comes with a wide range of emotions at different points in time. It is your right to feel any kind of emotion at any time and to express those emotions.

4. **You have the right to talk about your chronic illness and the feelings of grief that come with it.** Talking about your feelings of grief helps you understand them and, over time, helps you integrate them into your life. Find friends and family who are supportive of your feelings and will listen with empathy.

5. **You have the right to seek support from others.** Chronic illness may make you feel like you are battling alone, but everyone needs support from others. It is your right to ask for support from others when you need it. Seek out people who will make you feel supported without inhibiting your independence. It is OK to ask for help when you need it.

6. **You have the right to ask "why."** It is your right to wonder why you have a chronic illness. It is natural to wonder why this has happened to you and to explore all of the questions you may have. Why did this happen now? Why do I have to feel sick? Why would this happen to me?

7. **You have the right to speak up for your body and health.** It is your right to be in charge of how you take care of your body. You have the right to talk to your healthcare providers about how you want to manage your treatment. Your body and health are under your care, and you know best what works for you.

8. **You have the right to participate in any activity you want to.** As long as you are safe and able to participate, it is your right to do whatever you feel your body and health can handle. Don't let others tell you what you are and aren't able to do. As long as your doctor signs off, you can participate in many different activities. Travel, play sports, venture out into the world—do what makes your heart happy!

9. **You have the right to educate others about your illness.** It can be dangerous if others around you are unaware of the realities of your illness. To keep yourself safe and to create understanding about your illness, you have the right and the responsibility to educate others about your condition and your needs.

10. **You have the right to live fully.** Living with chronic illness does not stop you from living a full life. You can still live each day to its fullest and love the life you have. Although your chronic illness may limit you in some ways, there is always a way to find life and love in every moment.

ALSO BY ALAN WOLFELT

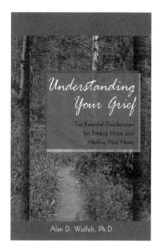

The Ten Essential Touchstones:

1. Open to the presence of your loss.
2. Dispel misconceptions about grief.
3. Embrace the uniqueness of your grief.
4. Explore your feelings of loss.
5. Recognize you are not crazy.
6. Understand the six needs of mourning.
7. Nurture yourself.
8. Reach out for help.
9. Seek reconciliation, not resolution.
10. Appreciate your transformation.

Understanding Your Grief
Ten Essential Touchstones for Finding Hope and Healing Your Heart

One of North America's leading grief educators, Dr. Alan Wolfelt has written many books about healing in grief. This book is his most comprehensive, covering the essential lessons that mourners have taught him in his three decades of working with the bereaved.

In compassionate, down-to-earth language, *Understanding Your Grief* describes ten touchstones—or trail markers—that are essential physical, emotional, cognitive, social, and spiritual signs for mourners to look for on their journey through grief.

Think of your grief as a wilderness—a vast, inhospitable forest. You must journey through this wilderness. To find your way out, you must become acquainted with its terrain and learn to follow the sometimes hard-to-find trail that leads to healing. In the wilderness of your grief, the touchstones are your trail markers. They are the signs that let you know you are on the right path. When you learn to identify and rely on the touchstones, you will find your way to hope and healing.

ISBN 978-1-879651-35-7 • 176 pages
softcover • $14.95

Companion
PRESS

All Dr. Wolfelt's publications can be ordered by mail from:
Companion Press
3735 Broken Bow Road
Fort Collins, CO 80526
(970) 226-6050
www.centerforloss.com

ALSO BY ALAN WOLFELT

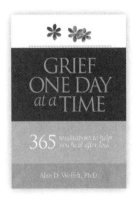

Grief One Day at a Time
365 Meditations to Help You Heal After Loss

After a loved one dies, each day can be a struggle. But each day, you can also find comfort and understanding in this daily companion. With one brief entry for every day of the calendar year, this little book by beloved grief counselor Dr. Alan Wolfelt offers small, one-day-at-a-time doses of guidance and healing.

ISBN 978-1-61722-238- 2 • 384 pages • softcover • $14.95

"This is a fabulous little meditation for those who are grieving. Our bereavement teams at Sangre de Cristo Hospice utilize this in our bereavement groups."
— Amazon reviewer

"The best daily reader on grief that I have found."
— Amazon reviewer

"I love this book so much! I recently lost my father to a brutal disease, too early in his senior life. This book has been so helpful for me. Having this book to turn to on a daily basis is helping me cope. I would be a lot more lost without this book."
— Amazon reviewer

"Very nice book with short, less than five-minute daily meditations for anyone who is suffering the loss of a loved one. Highly recommend!"
— Amazon reviewer

Companion
PRESS

All Dr. Wolfelt's publications can be ordered by mail from:
Companion Press
3735 Broken Bow Road
Fort Collins, CO 80526
(970) 226-6050
www.centerforloss.com

ALSO BY ALAN WOLFELT

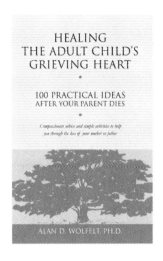

Healing the Adult Child's Grieving Heart
100 Practical Ideas

Offering heartfelt and simple advice, this book provides realistic suggestions and relief for an adult child whose parent has died. Practical advice is presented in a one-topic-per-page format that does not overwhelm but instead provides small, immediate ways for the reader to understand and embrace their grief.

ISBN 978-1-879651-31-9 • 128 pages
softcover • $11.95

"I bought this book shortly after my father passed away, and thought it was so good I ordered more copies for my siblings. This book is divided into subjects with text limited to one page per topic. While normally I like more detail, the author knows that in times of grief the brain more readily accepts smaller bits of information. I usually read one or two pages at a time. I also think this book would be very helpful to anyone regardless of religious beliefs."

— Amazon reviewer

"This is a must for anyone who has lost a parent. My book is marked, bent, and goes with me everywhere. I am new to grieving, and I find this a helpful guide toward healing."

— Amazon reviewer

"Simple, relevant, and gentle. I ordered one for my brother and sister to ease us into dialogue. Thank you, Dr. Wolfelt."

— Anne Chapman

Companion
PRESS

All Dr. Wolfelt's publications can be ordered by mail from:
Companion Press
3735 Broken Bow Road
Fort Collins, CO 80526
(970) 226-6050
www.centerforloss.com

ALSO BY ALAN WOLFELT

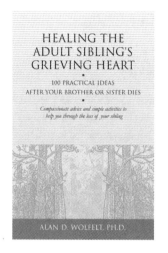

Healing the Adult Sibling's Grieving Heart
100 Practical Ideas After Your Brother or Sister Dies

Compassionate and heartfelt, this collection offers 100 practical ideas to help you understand and mourn the death of a sibling. The principles of grief and mourning are clearly defined, accompanied by action-oriented tips for embracing grief.

Whether a sibling has died as a young or older adult, whether the death was sudden or anticipated, this resource offers compassionate guidance for the normal and necessary journey through grief.

978-1-879651-29-6 • 128 pages • softcover • $11.95

"I was so grateful there was a book out there to help me in my grief when my brother died unexpectedly. The book let me know that it was OK to be sad, cry, and most of all to be easy on myself."
— Barbara Franklin

"At a time when I am hurting tremendously following the sudden, tragic death of my brother, this book has been a really wonderful source of validation and support. I like the fact that it's a very simple read, and that I can pick it up now and then and get a few helpful thoughts without spending a lot of time and energy. I even bought copies for my two sisters and sent them as gifts."
— Amazon reviewer

Companion
PRESS

All Dr. Wolfelt's publications can be ordered by mail from:
Companion Press
3735 Broken Bow Road
Fort Collins, CO 80526
(970) 226-6050
www.centerforloss.com

ALSO BY ALAN WOLFELT

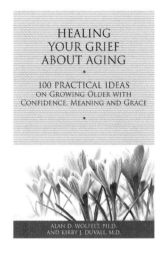

Healing Your Grief About Aging
100 Practical Ideas on Growing Older with Confidence, Meaning, and Grace

by Alan D. Wolfelt, Ph.D. and Kirby J. Duvall, M.D.

Getting older goes hand in hand with losses of many kinds—ending careers, empty nests, illness, the death of loved ones—and this book by one of the world's most beloved grief counselors helps readers acknowledge and mourn the many losses of aging while also offering advice for living better in older age.

The 100 practical tips and activities address the emotional, spiritual, cognitive, social, and physical needs of seniors who want to age authentically and gracefully. Whether you've just entered your 50s or are well on your way to the century mark, this book promises elder-friendly tips for comfort, laughter, and inspiration.

ISBN 978-1-61722-171-2 • 128 pages • softcover • $11.95

"This is a very easy read that can be helpful at different times of life. Alan Wolfelt has such a gift for teaching people how to look for the joy in life and guide them on the inevitable journey toward death."

— Amazon reviewer

Companion
PRESS

All Dr. Wolfelt's publications can be ordered by mail from:
Companion Press
3735 Broken Bow Road
Fort Collins, CO 80526
(970) 226-6050
www.centerforloss.com